# I.V. Therapy

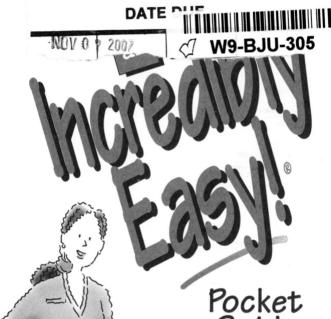

# Incredibly Easy!®

## Pocket Guide

LIPPINCOTT WILLIAMS & WILKINS
A Wolters Kluwer Company

Philadelphia • Baltimore • New York • London
Buenos Aires • Hong Kong • Sydney • Tokyo

## Staff

**Executive Publisher**
Judith A. Schilling McCann, RN, MSN

**Editorial Director**
David Moreau

**Clinical Director**
Joan M. Robinson, RN, MSN

**Senior Art Director**
Arlene Putterman

**Art Director**
Mary Ludwicki

**Editorial Project Manager**
Tracy S. Diehl

**Clinical Project Manager**
Beverly Ann Tscheschlog, RN, BS

**Editors**
Laura Bruck, Diane Labus, Brenna H. Mayer

**Clinical Editor**
Pamela Kovach, RN, BSN

**Copy Editors**
Kimberly Bilotta (supervisor), Tom DeZego,
Amy Furman, Pamela Wingrod

**Designer**
Lynn Foulk

**Illustrator**
Bot Roda

**Digital Composition Services**
Diane Paluba (manager), Joyce Rossi Biletz

**Manufacturing**
Patricia K. Dorshaw (director),
Beth J. Welsh

**Editorial Assistants**
Megan L. Aldinger, Karen J. Kirk,
Linda K. Ruhf

**Indexer**
Karen C. Comerford

IVIEPG010705 — D N O S A J
07 06 05      10 9 8 7 6 5 4 3 2 1

**Library of Congress Cataloging-in-Publication Data**
I.V. therapy : an incredibly easy pocket guide.
      p. ; cm.
   Includes bibliographical references and index.
1. Intravenous therapy — Handbooks, manuals, etc. I. Lippincott Williams & Wilkins. II.
Title: IV therapy. [DNLM: 1. Infusions,
Intravenous — Handbooks. WB 39 I935 2006]
RM170.I23 2006
615'.6 — dc22
ISBN 1-58255-435-8 (alk. paper)            2005006551

# Contents

Contributors and consultants     iv

Road map to I.V. therapy     v

| 1 | Fundamentals of I.V. therapy | 1 |
| 2 | Peripheral I.V. therapy | 27 |
| 3 | Central venous therapy | 77 |
| 4 | I.V. medications | 149 |
| 5 | Transfusions | 183 |
| 6 | Chemotherapy infusions | 221 |
| 7 | Parenteral nutrition | 259 |

## Appendices and index

The test zone     295

Selected references     307

Index     308

# Contributors and consultants

**Mary J. Dunn, ARNP,BC, MS**
Geriatric Nurse Practitioner
Adjunct Faculty
Florida Atlantic University
Geriatric Nurse Practitioner
Memory & Wellness Center and Christine E.
  Lynn College of Nursing
Boca Raton, Fla.

**Sandra Hamilton, RN, BSN, MEd, CRNI**
Critical Care Nurse
Kindred Hospital
Las Vegas

**Sue Masoorli, RN**
President/CEO
Perivascular Nurse Consultants, Inc.
Philadelphia

**Sharon D. O'Kelley, RN, OCN**
Clinical Nurse III
Duke University Hospital Systems
Durham, N.C.

**Susan Poole, BSN, MS, CRNI, CNSN**
Clinical Services
Option Care Inc.
Buffalo Grove, Ill.

**Nan Carey Riedé, RN, MSN**
Assistant Professor
Baptist College of Health Sciences
Memphis

**Christie Shelton, RN, MSN**
Nursing Instructor
Jacksonville (Ala.) State University

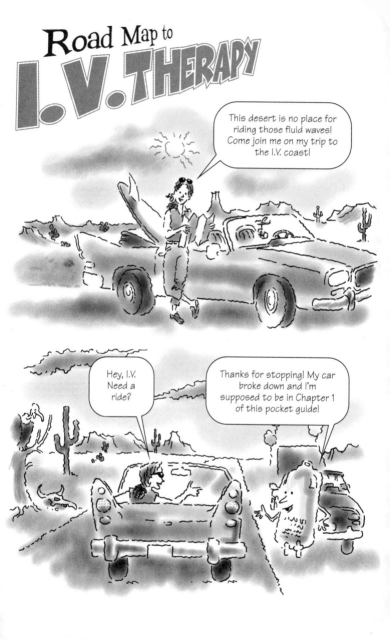

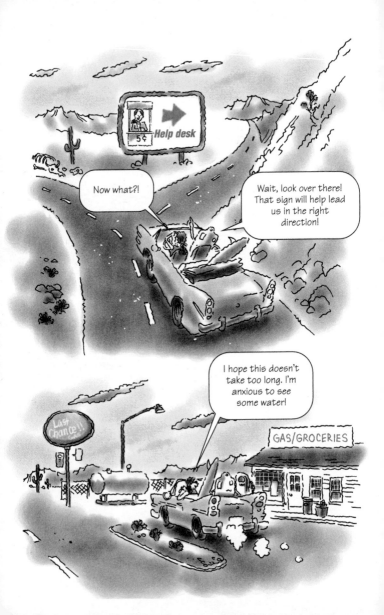

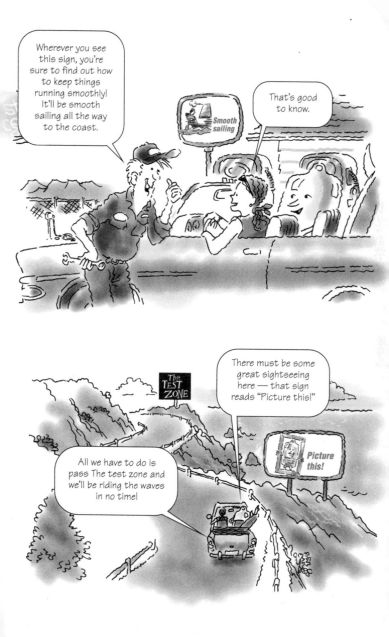

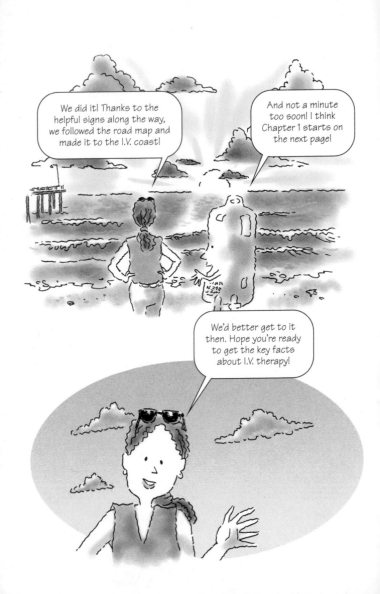

# Fundamentals of I.V. therapy

**1**

Don't gamble with I.V. therapy. Make sure you know these fundamentals!

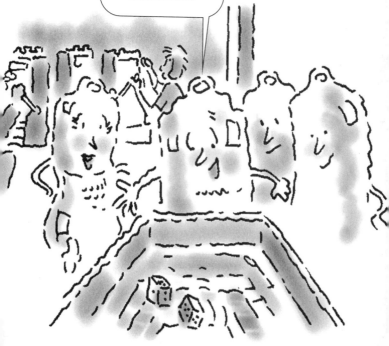

## Understanding electrolytes

Electrolyte concentrations are expressed in milliequivalents per liter (mEq/L) and milligrams per deciliter (mg/dl), as well as in International System (SI) units (mmol/L). Six major electrolytes play important roles in maintaining chemical balance:

 calcium

 chloride

 magnesium

 phosphorus

 potassium

 sodium.

# Calcium (Ca++)

- Major cation found in extracellular fluid of teeth and bones
- Normal serum level of 8.2 to 10.2 mg/dl (SI, 2.05 to 2.54 mmol/L)

## What to look for

### Hypercalcemia

- Anorexia
- Constipation
- Headache
- Hypertension
- Lethargy
- Muscle flaccidity
- Nausea
- Polydipsia
- Polyuria
- Vomiting

### Hypocalcemia

- Arrhythmias
- Bleeding
- Hypotension
- Muscle cramps
- Muscle tremor
- Paresthesia
- Tetany
- Tonic-clonic seizures

# Chloride (Cl⁻)

- Major anion found in extracellular fluid
- Normal serum level of 100 to 108 mEq/L (SI, 100 to 108 mmol/L)

## What to look for

### Hyperchloremia

- Dyspnea
- Fluid retention and pitting edema
- Hypertension
- Metabolic acidosis
  - Kussmaul's respirations
  - Lethargy
  - Tachycardia

### Hypochloremia

- Decreased respirations
- Increased muscle excitability
  - Muscle cramps
  - Muscle twitching
  - Muscle weakness
- Tetany

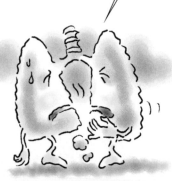

Decreased (gasp!) respirations are never a good sign!

# Magnesium (Mg++)

- Major cation found in intracellular fluid (closely related to calcium and potassium)
- Normal serum level of 1.3 to 2.1 mg/dl (SI, 0.65 to 1.05 mmol/L) with 33% bound protein and remainder as free cations

## What to look for

### Hypermagnesemia

- Arrhythmias
- Coma
- Drowsiness
- Hypotension
- Lethargy
- Slow, weak pulse
- Vague GI symptoms (such as nausea)
- Vague neuromuscular changes (such as tremor)

### Hypomagnesemia

- Anorexia
- Arrhythmias
- Confusion
- Dizziness
- Hyperirritability
- Leg and foot cramps
- Nausea
- Seizures
- Tremor
- Vasomotor changes

# Phosphorus (P)

- Major anion found in intracellular fluid
- Normal serum level (phosphate level) of 2.7 to 4.5 mg/dl (SI, 0.87 to 1.45 mmol/L)

## What to look for

### Hyperphosphatemia

- Anorexia
- Arrhythmias and muscle twitching with sudden rise in phosphate level
- Decreased mental status
- Hyperreflexia
- Nausea and vomiting
- Paresthesia
- Renal failure
- Tetany
- Vague neuroexcitability to tetany and seizures

### Hypophosphatemia

- Anorexia
- Lethargy
- Malaise
- Muscle weakness
- Myalgia
- Paresthesia (circumoral and peripheral)
- Severe hypophosphatemia
  - Cardiomyopathy
  - Cyanosis
  - Decreased cardiac output
  - Hypotension
  - Respiratory failure
  - Rhabdomyolysis
- Speech defects (such as stuttering or stammering)

# Potassium (K+)

- Major cation in intracellular fluid
- Normal serum level of 3.5 to 5 mEq/L (SI, 3.5 to 5 mmol/L)

## What to look for

### Hyperkalemia

- Diarrhea
- Muscle weakness
- Nausea
- Oliguria

### Hypokalemia

- Decreased blood pressure
- Decreased GI, skeletal muscle, and cardiac muscle function
- Decreased reflexes
- Muscle weakness or irritability
- Nausea and vomiting
- Paralytic ileus
- Rapid, weak, irregular pulse

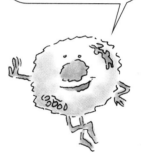

Potassium is a major cation in my intracellular fluid. It isn't pretty when I get too little or too much!

# Sodium (Na⁺)

- Major cation in extracellular fluid
- Normal serum level of 135 to 145 mEq/L (SI, 135 to 145 mmol/L)

## What to look for

### Hypernatremia

- Agitation
- Confusion
- Fever
- Flushed skin
- Lethargy
- Hypervolemia
  - Bounding pulse
  - Dyspnea
  - Hypertension
- Hypovolemia
  - Dry mucous membranes
  - Oliguria
  - Orthostatic hypotension
- Thirst
- Twitching
- Weakness

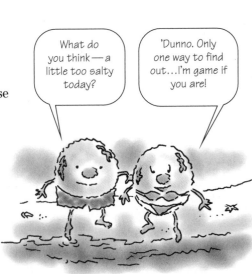

### Hyponatremia

- Abdominal cramps
- Altered level of consciousness
- Decreased skin turgor
- Headache
- Muscle weakness
- Nausea
- Seizures
- Tremor

# Identifying fluid imbalances

By carefully assessing a patient before and during I.V. therapy, you can identify fluid imbalances early — before serious complications develop.

## What to look for

### Fluid deficit

- Decreased central venous pressure
- Decreased salivation
- Difficulty forming words (patient may moisten mouth before beginning to speak)
- Diminished blood pressure, commonly with orthostatic hypotension
- Diminished urine output
- Dry, cracked lips
- Furrows in tongue
- Increased blood urea nitrogen (BUN) levels
- Increased hematocrit
- Increased serum electrolyte levels
- Increased serum osmolarity
- Increased, thready pulse rate
- Lack of moisture in groin and axillae
- Mental status changes
- Poor skin turgor (not a reliable sign in elderly patients)
- Sunken eyes, dry conjunctivae, decreased tearing
- Thirst
- Weakness
- Weight loss

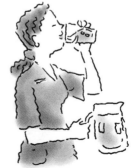

Thirst…(gulp)…is a key sign of fluid deficit! Now excuse me as I replenish!

## Fluid excess

- Bounding pulse that isn't easily obliterated
- Decreased BUN levels
- Decreased hematocrit
- Decreased serum electrolyte levels
- Dyspnea
- Edema of dependent body parts; sacral edema in patients on bed rest
- Elevated blood pressure
- Fuller-than-normal cheeks
- Increased respiratory rate
- Jugular vein distention
- Moist crackles or rhonchi on auscultation
- Periorbital edema
- Puffy eyelids
- Reduced serum osmolarity
- Slow emptying of hand veins when the arm is raised
- Weight gain

# Understanding I.V. solutions

There are three basic types of I.V. solutions:

 isotonic

 hypertonic

 hypotonic.

 *Picture this!*

## Understanding I.V. solutions

Solution type depends on whether you want to change or maintain a patient's body fluid status.

**Isotonic solution**
Because an isotonic solution stays in the intravascular space, it expands the intravascular compartment.

**Hypertonic solution**
A hypertonic solution draws fluid into the intravascular compartment from the cells and the interstitial compartments.

**Hypotonic solution**
A hypotonic solution shifts fluid out of the intravascular compartment, hydrating the cells and the interstitial compartments.

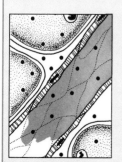
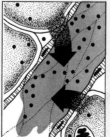
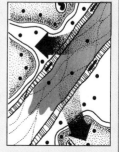

## Isotonic solutions

- Osmolarity about equal to that of serum
- Expand the intravascular compartment

### Examples

- 5% albumin (308 mOsm/L)
- Dextrose 5% in water ($D_5W$) (260 mOsm/L)
- Hetastarch (310 mOsm/L)
- Lactated Ringer's (275 mOsm/L)
- Normal saline (308 mOsm/L)
- Normosol (295 mOsm/L)
- Ringer's (275 mOsm/L)

### What to do

- Closely monitor the patient for signs of fluid overload, especially if he's hypertensive or at risk for heart failure.

### What to consider

- Lactated Ringer's contraindicated if the patient's blood pH is greater than 7.5 because liver converts lactate to bicarbonate
- $D_5W$ contraindicated in patients at risk for increased intracranial pressure (ICP) because it acts like a hypotonic solution, thereby shifting more fluid into the cells and interstitial compartments, raising ICP more

# Hypertonic solutions

- Osmolarity higher than that of serum
- Draw fluid into the intravascular compartment from the cells and the interstitial compartments

## Examples

- 3% sodium chloride (1,025 mOsm/L)
- 7.5% sodium chloride (2,400 mOsm/L)
- 25% albumin (1,500 mOsm/L)
- Dextrose 5% in half-normal saline (406 mOsm/L)
- Dextrose 5% in lactated Ringer's (575 mOsm/L)
- Dextrose 5% in normal saline (560 mOsm/L)

## What to do

- Closely monitor the patient receiving a hypertonic solution for circulatory overload.

## What to consider

- Contraindicated in patients with conditions that cause cellular dehydration such as diabetic ketoacidosis
- Contraindicated in patients with impaired heart or kidney function because of possible fluid overload

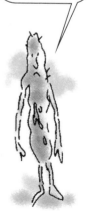

If I knew this is what they meant by a hypertonic liquid diet, I never would have agreed to it.

# Hypotonic solutions

- Osmolarity lower than that of serum
- Shift fluid out of the intravascular compartment
- Hydrate the cells and the interstitial compartments

## Examples

- 0.33% sodium chloride (103 mOsm/L)
- Dextrose 2.5% in water (126 mOsm/L)
- Half-normal saline (154 mOsm/L)

## What to do

- Administer hypotonic solutions cautiously because they can cause cardiovascular collapse from intravascular fluid depletion and increased ICP from fluid shift into brain cells.

## What to consider

- Contraindicated in patients at risk for increased ICP from stroke, head trauma, or neurosurgery
- Contraindicated in patients at risk for third-space fluid shifts, such as those with burns, trauma, or low serum protein levels from malnutrition or liver disease

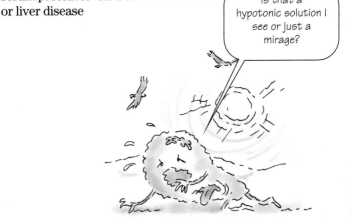

Is that a hypotonic solution I see or just a mirage?

## Comparing I.V. delivery methods

## Direct injection into a vein

- Commonly referred to as an *I.V. push*
- Generally doesn't involve an administration site
- Indicated when a nonirritating drug with a low risk of immediate adverse reactions is required for a patient with no other I.V. needs

### The pros

- Eliminates the risk of complications from an indwelling venipuncture device
- Eliminates the inconvenience of an indwelling venipuncture device

### The cons

- Can only be given by a doctor or specially certified nurse
- Requires venipuncture
- Requires two syringes
- Infiltration risk
- Impossible to dilute the drug
- Impossible to interrupt delivery when irritation occurs
- Risks clotting with drug administration of even a small volume over a long period

# Direct injection through an existing infusion line

- Indicated when a drug is incompatible with the I.V. solution and must be given as a bolus injection for therapeutic effect
- Indicated when the patient requires immediate high blood levels of a medication
- Indicated in emergencies, when the drug must be given quickly for immediate effect

## The pros

- Doesn't require additional venipuncture
- Doesn't require needle puncture
- Allows the use of an I.V. solution to test venipuncture device patency before administration
- Allows continued venous access in case of adverse reactions
- Reduces the risk of infiltration with irritating drugs

## The cons

- Increases the risk of incompatibility with drugs administered by piggyback infusion
- Restricts patient mobility
- Increases the risk of undetected infiltration because slow infusion makes it difficult to see swelling in the infiltration area
- Increases the risk of phlebitis or vein irritation from an increased number of drugs

# Intermittent infusion using the piggyback method

- Commonly used with drugs given over short periods at varying intervals

## The pros

- Avoids multiple I.M. injections
- Permits repeated administration of drugs through a single I.V. line
- Provides high drug blood levels for short periods without causing drug toxicity

## The cons

- May cause periods when the drug level becomes too low to be clinically effective

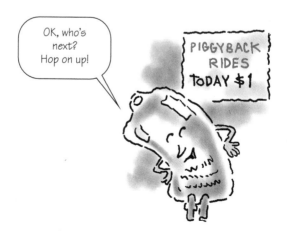

# Intermittent infusion using a saline lock

- Indicated when the patient requires constant venous access but not continuous infusion

### The pros

- Provides venous access for patients with fluid restrictions
- Allows better patient mobility between doses
- Preserves veins by reducing frequent venipuncture
- Lowers the cost of the infusion

### The cons

- Requires close monitoring during administration so the device can be flushed on completion

# Intermittent infusion using a volume-control set

- Has a medication chamber that allows delivery of small doses over an extended period
- Indicated when the patient requires a low volume of fluid

### The pros

- Requires only one large-volume container and prevents fluid overload from runaway infusion

### The cons

- May have high equipment costs
- Carries a high contamination risk
- Requires that the flow clamp be closed when the set empties, if the set doesn't contain a membrane that blocks the air passage when it's empty

# Continuous infusion through a primary line

- Indicated when continuous serum levels are needed

## The pros

- Maintains steady serum levels
- Lowers the risk of rapid shock and vein irritation from a large volume of fluid diluting the drug

## The cons

- Increases the risk of incompatibility with drugs administered by piggyback infusion
- Restricts patient mobility when the patient is connected to an I.V. system
- Increases the risk of undetected infiltration because a slow infusion rate makes it difficult to see swelling in the infiltration area

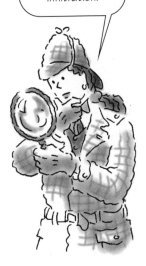

A slow infusion rate makes it difficult to detect infiltration.

# Continuous infusion through a secondary line

- Indicated when the patient requires a continuous infusion of two or more compatible admixtures administered at different rates
- Indicated when there's a moderate-to-high chance of abruptly stopping one admixture without infusing the drug remaining in the I.V. tubing

## The pros

- Permits the primary infusion and each secondary infusion to be given at different rates
- Permits the primary line to be shut off but kept standing by to maintain venous access in case a secondary line must be abruptly stopped

## The cons

- Eliminates the use of drugs with immediate incompatibility
- Increases the risk of phlebitis or vein irritation from an increased number of drugs
- Uses multiple I.V. systems, which can create physical barriers to patient care and limit patient mobility

## Calculating infusion flow rates

Volume control devices and the correct administration technique help prevent complications.

### Macrodrip
- Delivers 10, 15, or 20 gtt/ml

### Microdrip
- Delivers 60 gtt/ml

*Help desk*

5¢

### Reading an I.V. order

Orders for I.V. therapy may be standardized for different illnesses and therapies, such as burn treatment, or individualized for a particular patient. Some facility policies dictate an automatic stop order for I.V. fluids. For example, I.V. orders are good for 24 hours from the time they're written, unless otherwise specified.

**It's complete**
A complete order for I.V. therapy should specify:
- type and amount of therapy
- additives and their concentrations (such as 10 mEq potassium chloride in 500 ml dextrose 5% in water)
- rate and volume of infusion
- duration of infusion.

**When it isn't complete**
If you find that an order isn't complete or you think an I.V. order is inappropriate because of the patient's condition, consult the doctor.

## Calculating flow rates

Remember that the number of drops required to deliver 1 ml varies with the type of administration set used and its manufacturer:

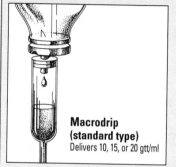

**Macrodrip (standard type)**
Delivers 10, 15, or 20 gtt/ml

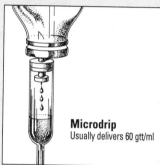

**Microdrip**
Usually delivers 60 gtt/ml

• Manufacturers calibrate their devices differently; look for the "drip factor" — expressed in drops per milliliter, or gtt/ml — in the packaging that accompanies the set you're using.
• When you know your device's drip factor, use the following formula to calculate specific flow rates:

$$\frac{\text{volume of infusion (in milliliters)}}{\text{time of infusion (in minutes)}} \times \text{drip factor (in drops per milliliter)} =$$

flow rate (in drops per minute)

• After you calculate the flow rate for the set you're using, remove your watch or position your wrist so you can look at your watch and the drops at the same time.
• Adjust the clamp to achieve the ordered flow rate, and count the drops for 1 full minute.
• Readjust the clamp as necessary, and count the drops for another minute.
• Keep adjusting the clamp and counting the drops until you have the correct rate.

## Documenting I.V. therapy

Documentation provides:
- accurate description of care
- record of what the patient received to help with continuing care
- record for health care insurers of equipment and supplies used.

## Documenting initiation of I.V. therapy

When documenting the insertion of a venipuncture device or the beginning of therapy, specify:
- size and type of the device
- name of the person who inserted the device
- date and time
- site location
- type of solution
- additives
- flow rate
- use of an electric infusion pump or other type of flow controller
- complications, patient response, and nursing interventions
- patient teaching and evidence of patient understanding
- number of attempts (successful and unsuccessful).

### How to label an I.V. bag

When you place the label on an I.V. bag, be sure not to cover the name of the I.V. solution. To properly label an I.V solution container, include the:
- patient's name, identification number, and room number
- date and time the container was hung
- additives and their amounts
- rate at which the solution is to run
- sequential container number
- expiration date and time of infusion.

## Documenting I.V. therapy maintenance

When documenting I.V. therapy maintenance, specify:
- condition of the site
- site care provided
- dressing changes
- site changes
- tubing and solution changes
- your teaching and evidence of patient understanding.

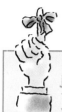

**Memory jogger**

To remind yourself of the need to check and adjust flow rates, remember this tongue twister:

*Fight fickle flow with frequent follow-up.*

## Documenting discontinuation of I.V. therapy

When you document the discontinuation of I.V. therapy, specify:
- time and date
- reason for discontinuing therapy
- assessment of venipuncture site before and after the venous access device is removed
- complications, patient reactions, and nursing interventions
- integrity of the venous access device on removal
- follow-up actions, such as applying an adhesive bandage to the site and restarting the I.V. infusion in another extremity.

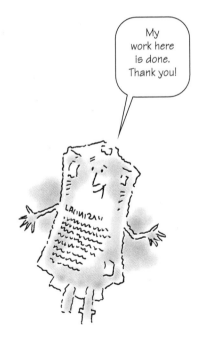

# Peripheral I.V. therapy

# 2

Check out these steps on the where, what, how, and why of peripheral I.V. therapy.

Ah, the sites and sounds of peripheral I.V. therapy. Boy, that takes me back!

## Comparing peripheral venipuncture sites

### Digital veins

- Run along the lateral and dorsal portions of the fingers

#### The pros

- May be used for short-term therapy
- May be used when other means aren't available

#### The cons

- Requires splinting fingers with a tongue blade, which decreases patient's ability to use his hand
- Uncomfortable for the patient
- Significant risk of infiltration
- Not used if the veins in the dorsum of the hand are already used

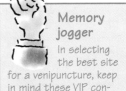

**Memory jogger**

In selecting the best site for a venipuncture, keep in mind these VIP considerations:

Vein — location, condition, and physical path along the extremity

Infusion — purpose and duration

Patient — degree of cooperation and compliance as well as his preference

**Picture this!**

## Commonly used veins

Veins of the arms and fingers are commonly used in peripheral I.V. therapy.

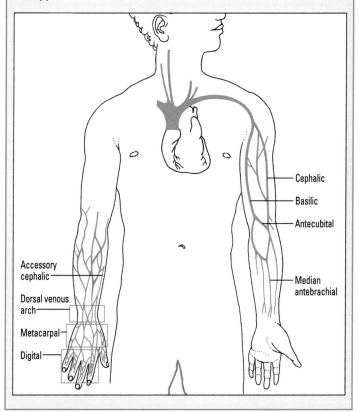

## Metacarpal veins

- Located on the dorsum of the hand
- Formed by the union of the digital veins between the knuckles

### The pros

- Easily accessible
- Lie flat on the back of the hand
- More difficult to dislodge needle or catheter
- Natural splinting achieved by bones of the hand in an adult or large child

### The cons

- Wrist movement decreased unless a short catheter is used
- Painful insertion likely because of the large number of nerve endings in the hands
- Phlebitis likely at the site

Metacarpal veins can be found on the back of the hand.

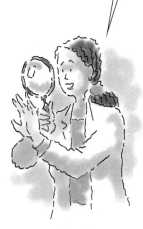

# Dorsal venous network

- Located on the dorsal portion of the arm

## The pros
- Splinted by the metacarpal veins, making access easier

## The cons
- May be difficult to see or find the vein
- May be difficult to access in elderly patients because of poor skin turgor
- Difficult for the patient to write or eat with the device in place, especially if it's placed in the patient's dominant arm
- Requires a stabilization device

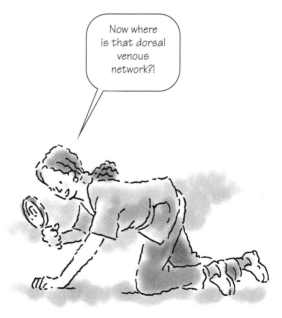

Now where is that dorsal venous network?!

# Median antebrachial vein

- Arises from the palm
- Runs along the ulnar side of the forearm

## The pros

- Holds winged needles well
- Last resort when no other means available

## The cons

- Painful insertion or infiltration damage possible because of the many nerve endings in the area
- High risk of infiltration

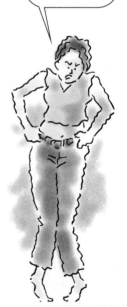

Use a median antebrachial vein as a last resort. Kind of like my plan for wearing these jeans.

# Accessory cephalic vein

- Runs along the radial bone as a continuation of the metacarpal veins of the thumb

## The pros

- Large vein excellent for venipuncture
- Readily accepts large-gauge needles
- Doesn't impair mobility
- Doesn't require an arm board in an older child or adult

## The cons

- Some difficulty positioning the catheter flush with the skin
- Discomfort during movement due to the location of the device at the bend of the wrist

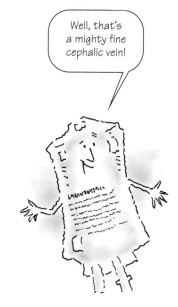

Well, that's a mighty fine cephalic vein!

# Antecubital veins

- Located in the antecubital fossa (median cephalic, on radial side; median basilic, on ulnar side; median cubital, which rises in front of the elbow joint)

### The pros

- Large vein, which facilitates drawing blood
- Commonly visible or palpable in children when other veins won't dilate
- May be used in an emergency

### The cons

- Difficult to splint the elbow area with an arm board
- Veins possibly small and scarred if blood has been drawn frequently from this site

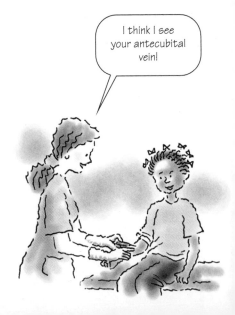

# Basilic vein

- Runs along the ulnar side of the forearm and upper arm

## The pros

- Readily accepts large-gauge needles
- Straight, strong vein suitable for venipuncture

## The cons

- Uncomfortable position for the patient during insertion
- Painful insertion because of penetration of the dermal layer of the skin, where nerve endings are located
- Vein stabilization possibly difficult

# Cephalic vein

- Runs along the radial side of the forearm and upper arm

## The pros
- Large vein excellent for venipuncture
- Readily accepts large-gauge needles

## The cons
- Decreased joint movement due to the proximity of the device to the elbow
- Vein stabilization possibly difficult

## Comparing venipuncture devices

## Over-the-needle catheter

### Why it's done
• To provide long-term therapy for an active or agitated patient

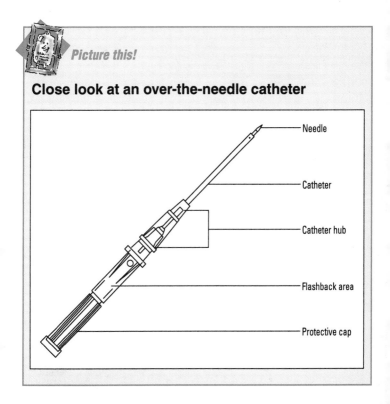

*Picture this!*

**Close look at an over-the-needle catheter**

Needle

Catheter

Catheter hub

Flashback area

Protective cap

## The pros

- Inadvertent puncture of vein less likely than with a winged steel needle set
- More comfortable for the patient
- Radiopaque thread for easy location
- Attached syringe (available with some units) that permits easy check of blood return and prevents air from entering the vessel on insertion
- Activity-restricting device, such as an arm board, rarely required

## The cons

- Difficult to insert
- Extra care required to ensure that the needle and catheter are inserted into the vein

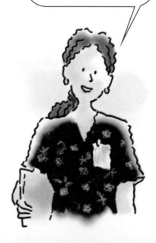

An over-the-needle catheter may be more comfortable for the patient but may be difficult to insert.

# Winged steel needle set

## Why it's done

- To provide short-term therapy for a cooperative adult patient
- To provide therapy of any duration for an infant or child
- To provide therapy of any duration for an elderly patient with fragile or sclerotic veins
- To give a single-dose administration

## The pros

- Thin-walled, extremely sharp needle
- Ideal for I.V. push drugs
- Available with a catheter that can be left in place, such as an over-the-needle catheter

## The cons

- Infiltration easily caused if a rigid needle winged infusion device is used

*Picture this!*

## Close look at a winged steel needle set

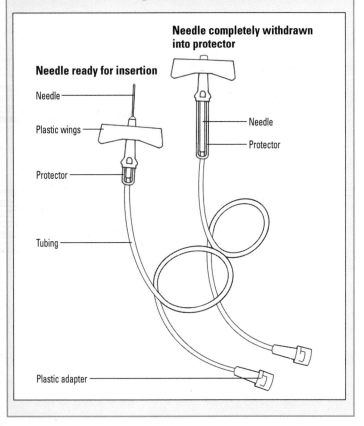

## Comparing needle and catheter gauges

| Gauge | Uses | Nursing considerations |
|---|---|---|
| *16* | • Adolescents and adults<br>• Major surgery<br>• Trauma<br>• Whenever large amounts of fluids must be infused | • Painful insertion<br>• Requires large vein |
| *18* | • Older children, adolescents, and adults<br>• Administration of blood and blood components and other viscous infusions | • Painful insertion<br>• Requires large vein |
| *20* | • Children, adolescents, and adults<br>• Suitable for most I.V. infusions, including blood, blood components, and other viscous solutions | • Commonly used |
| *22* | • Infants, toddlers, children, adolescents, and adults (especially elderly)<br>• Suitable for most I.V. infusions | • Easier to insert into small, thin, fragile veins<br>• Slower flow rates must be maintained<br>• Difficult to insert into tough skin |
| *24, 26* | • Neonates, infants, toddlers, school-age children, adolescents, and adults (especially elderly)<br>• Suitable for most infusions, but flow rates are slower | • For extremely small veins — for example, small veins of fingers or veins of inner arms in elderly patients<br>• Possibly difficult to insert into tough skin |

## Performing venipuncture

## Dilating the vein

### Why it's done
- To trap blood in the vein
- To better visualize the vein

### What to do
- Place the arm in a dependent position to increase capillary flow.
- Apply a tourniquet.
- Instruct the patient to open and close his fist several times to distend the vein.
- Leave the tourniquet on for no longer than 2 minutes to prevent bruising.

## Preparing the site

### Why it's done

- To prevent infection and avoid introducing organisms into the blood

### What to do

- Wash your hands and put on gloves.
- Clip—not shave—the hairs around the site, if necessary.
- Clean the site with chlorhexidine.
- Use a vigorous back-and-forth motion to clean the site.
- Allow the site to dry thoroughly before insertion.

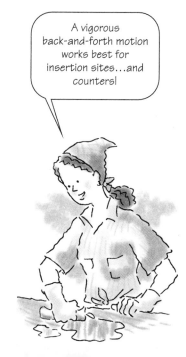

# Using a local anesthetic

## Why it's done
- To reduce the discomfort of venipuncture

## What to do
- Review the patient's record for possible allergies.
- Describe the procedure to the patient.
- Administer the local anesthetic.

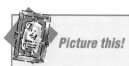

*Picture this!*

## Administering a local anesthetic

To administer a local anesthetic, follow these steps:
- Use a U-100 insulin syringe with a 27G needle.
- Draw 0.1 ml of 1% lidocaine without epinephrine.
- Clean the venipuncture site.
- Insert the needle next to the vein.
- Introduce about one-third of the needle into the skin at a 30-degree angle.
- If the vein is deep, inject the lidocaine over the top of it.
- Aspirate for a blood return to make sure you don't inject lidocaine into the vein.
- Hold your thumb on the plunger of the syringe during insertion to avoid unnecessary movement after the needle is under the skin.
- Without aspirating, quickly inject the lidocaine until a small wheal appears, as shown below.
- Quickly withdraw the syringe.
- Massage the wheal with an alcohol swab to make the wheal disappear but the vein visible.
- Instruct the patient that skin numbness will last about 30 minutes.
- Insert the venipuncture device into the vein.

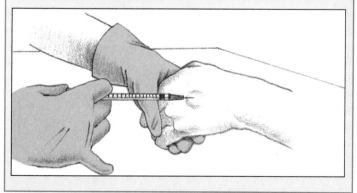

# Stabilizing veins

### Antecubital fossa
- Tell the patient to form a tight fist and fully extend his arm.
- Anchor the skin with your thumb, 2″ to 3″ (5 to 7.5 cm) below the antecubital fossa.

### Basilic vein at outer arm
- Tell the patient to make a tight fist and flex his elbow.
- While standing behind the flexed arm, retract the skin away from the site, and anchor the vein with your thumb.
- As an alternative, rotate the patient's extended lower arm inward, and approach the vein from behind the arm. (This position may be difficult for the patient to maintain.)

### Cephalic vein above wrist
- Tell the patient to make a tight fist.
- Stretch his fist laterally downward.
- Immobilize the skin with the thumb of your other hand.

### Inner arm
- Extend the patient's closed fist backward from the wrist.
- Anchor the vein with your thumb above the wrist.

### Inner aspect of wrist
- Extend the patient's open hand backward from the wrist.
- Anchor the vein with your thumb below the insertion site.

### Hand veins
- Stretch the patient's hand and wrist downward.
- Hold the skin taut with your thumb.

## Inserting an I.V. catheter

To insert an I.V. catheter, follow these steps:
• Tell the patient that you're about to insert the device.
• Hold the needle bevel up and enter the skin directly over the vein at a 5- to 15-degree angle.
• Push the needle directly through the skin and into the vein in one motion.
• Check the flash chamber for blood return.
• Level the insertion device slightly and advance the device to at least half its length to make sure that the cannula has entered the vein.
• Grasp the cannula hub to hold it in the vein and withdraw the needle.
• Press lightly on the catheter tip to prevent bleeding as you withdraw the needle.
• Advance the cannula up to the hub.

If you follow these steps, inserting an I.V. catheter can be a piece of cake...or in my case, a piece of pie!

## Obtaining a blood sample

- Place a pad underneath the site to protect the bed linens.
- Remove the inner needle if you're using an over-the-needle device, after the venipuncture device is correctly placed.
- Leave the tourniquet tied.
- Attach the syringe to the venipuncture device's hub.
- Withdraw the appropriate amount of blood.
- Release the tourniquet and disconnect the syringe.
- Quickly attach the saline lock or I.V. tubing.
- Regulate the flow rate.
- Stabilize the device.
- Insert the blood into the evacuated tubes, with a 19G needle-less device attached to the syringe.
- Complete I.V. line placement.

## Maintaining peripheral I.V. therapy

## Methods for taping an I.V. site

### Chevron method

- Cut a long strip of ½″ tape.
- Place the tape sticky side up under the hub of the catheter.
- Cross the ends of the tape over the hub.
- Secure the tape to the patient's skin on the opposite sides of the hub.
- Apply a piece of 1″ tape across the two wings of the chevron.
- Loop the tubing.
- Secure it with another piece of 1″ tape.
- Apply a label with the date and time of insertion, type and gauge of the needle, and your initials.

### U method

- Cut a strip of 1¼″ tape.
- Place the tape, sticky side up, under the hub of the catheter.
- Bring each side of the tape up, folding it over the wings of the catheter.
- Press it down, parallel to the hub.

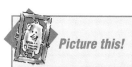

**Picture this!**

### Taping techniques

If you use tape to secure the venipuncture device to the insertion site, use one of these methods.

**Chevron method**

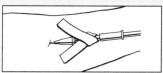

**U method**

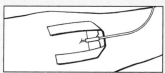

**H method**

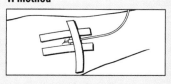

- Apply tape to stabilize the catheter.
- Apply a label with the date and time of insertion, type and gauge of the catheter, and your initials.

## H method

- Cut three strips of 1″ tape.
- Place one strip of tape over each wing, keeping the tape parallel to the catheter.
- Place the third strip of tape perpendicular to the first two.
- Put the tape directly on top of the wings.
- Make sure that the catheter is secure.
- Apply a dressing.
- Apply a label with the date and time of insertion, type and gauge of the catheter, and your initials.

# Applying a transparent semipermeable dressing

## Why it's done
- To prevent infection
- To secure the venipuncture device

## What to do
- Make sure that the insertion site is clean and dry.
- Remove the dressing from the package.
- Using aseptic technique, remove the protective seal.
- Avoid touching the sterile surface.
- Place the dressing directly over the insertion site and the hub.
- Avoid covering the tubing.
- Avoid stretching the dressing; doing so may cause itching.
- Tuck the dressing around and under the catheter hub to make the site occlusive to microorganisms.
- To remove the dressing, grasp one corner, and then lift and stretch.

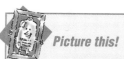

**Picture this!**

### Close look at applying a transparent semipermeable dressing

A transparent semipermeable dressing, shown below, allows visual assessment of the catheter insertion site.

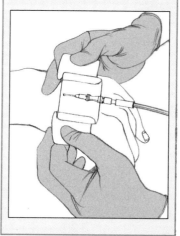

# Changing a peripheral I.V. dressing

## Why it's done
- To prevent infection
- To prevent compromising the integrity of the dressing

## What to do
- Wash your hands.
- Put on gloves.
- Hold the needle or catheter in place with your nondominant hand to prevent movement or dislodgment that could lead to infiltration.
- Gently remove the tape and the dressing.
- If you detect signs of infection, infiltration, or phlebitis, apply pressure to the area with a sterile gauze pad and remove the catheter or needle. Maintain pressure on the area until the bleeding stops. Apply a bandage. Using new equipment, insert the I.V. access device at another site.
- If you don't detect complications, hold the needle or catheter at the hub and carefully clean around the site with a chlorhexidine swab or alcohol pad, using a vigorous side-to-side motion.
- Allow the area to dry completely.
- Retape the device.
- Apply a transparent semipermeable dressing.
- Change the dressing at least every 72 hours, following your facility's policy.

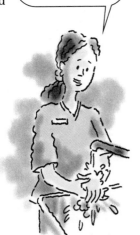

Proper hand washing is the first step in providing safe I.V. care to patients.

# Changing an administration set

## Why it's done

- To prevent infection or thrombophlebitis

## What to do

- Reduce the I.V. flow rate.
- Keeping the old spike upright and above the patient's heart level, insert the new spike into the I.V. container.
- Prime the system.
- Place a sterile gauze pad under the needle or hub of the plastic catheter to create a sterile field.
- Disconnect the old tubing from the venipuncture device, but don't dislodge or move the I.V. device.
- If you have trouble disconnecting the old tubing, use a pair of hemostats to hold the hub securely while twisting and removing the end of the tubing, or grasp the venipuncture device with one pair of hemostats and the hard plastic of the administration set's luer-lock end with another pair and pull the hemostats in opposite directions.
- Avoid clamping the hemostats shut; this may crack the tubing adapter or venipuncture device.
- Using aseptic technique, quickly attach the new primed tubing to the I.V. device.
- Adjust the flow to the prescribed rate.
- Label the new tubing with the date and time of the change.
- Change the administration set at least every 72 hours, following your facility's policy.

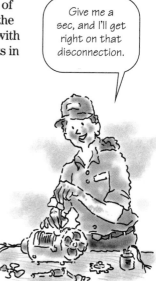

Give me a sec, and I'll get right on that disconnection.

# Infusing additive solutions

## Why it's done
- To administer additional solutions
- To maintain a primary line in case of adverse reactions to an additive

## What to do
To infuse two compatible solutions simultaneously, follow these steps:
- Use an add-a-line administration set.
- Connect an administration set with an attached needleless access catheter to the secondary solution container.
- Prime the tubing.
- Hang the container at the same level as the primary solution.
- Clean a Y-site in the lower part of the primary tubing, using a povidone-iodine or alcohol swab.
- Attach the secondary infusion set to the Y-site.
- Secure the secondary infusion set to the Y-site.
- Lower the primary infusion with the supplied extension hook below the level of the secondary container.
- Open the flow clamp of the secondary set and adjust the rate as prescribed. (Remember that with this setup, you don't have a back-check valve above the Y-site, so one solution may flow back into the other.)

*Picture this!*

## I.V. set-up for simultaneous infusion

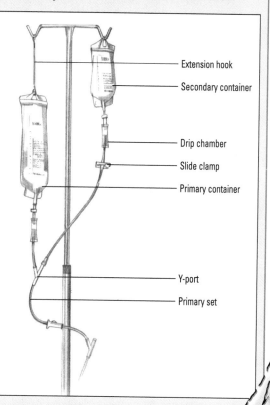

Extension hook

Secondary container

Drip chamber

Slide clamp

Primary container

Y-port

Primary set

## Managing patients with special needs

# I.V. therapy in pediatric patients

### What to do

- Palpate to ensure you have a vein — not an artery.
- If necessary, use clove-hitch and mummy restraints.
- Engage the parents' help to calm an infant or young child.
- Choose an appropriate venipuncture site.
  – In infants, the best sites include the hands, feet, antecubital fossa, dorsum of hand, and especially the scalp (scalp veins are most commonly used for infants younger than age 6 months).
  – In toddlers, dorsal foot veins and saphenous veins in the leg may be used, but dorsal hand veins allow the greatest mobility.
- Don't use a tourniquet or rubber band on a scalp vein. If you need a tourniquet effect, tip the infant's head down to facilitate filling of the superficial veins. When you see a blood return (usually it will be slight), tip the infant back to a horizontal or vertical position.
- Insert the venous access device caudally to make stabilizing easier.
- For long-term and antibiotic therapy (when venous access is poor), use an over-the-needle catheter.

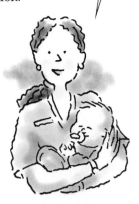

The best sites for I.V. insertion in infants include the head, hands, and feet.

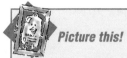

*Picture this!*

## Identifying scalp veins

Scalp veins are usually the best veins to use when administering I.V. therapy to an infant. The most commonly used veins are illustrated below.

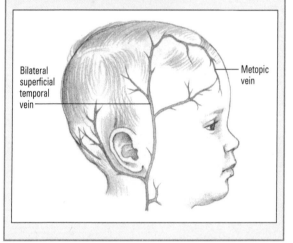

Bilateral superficial temporal vein

Metopic vein

- Tape the site as you would for an adult, so the skin over the access site is easily visible. Avoid overtaping, which makes inspecting the site and the surrounding tissues more difficult and may cause trauma when the device is removed.
- Cover the site with a stretch net, which can be easily rolled back for inspection.
- Protect the insertion site by taping a plastic medicine cup over it.

## What to consider

- In the scalp, arteries and veins may look similar. Remember, you'll feel a pulse with an artery.
- Consider using a topical or transdermal anesthetic to decrease the patient's discomfort.
- A small-diameter, winged over-the-needle catheter (commonly called a *scalp vein catheter*), which is less likely to cause traumatic injury to the vein, is always the preferred venous access device.
- The head veins most frequently used are the bilateral superficial temporal veins above the ear and the metopic vein running down the middle of the forehead.
- Scalp veins are extremely fragile and should be used only with infants younger than age 6 months; an older child is more likely to move his head and dislodge the venipuncture device.

# I.V. therapy in elderly patients

## What to do

- Choose the appropriate venipuncture site.
- Use a winged steel needle, the preferred venous access device, because it's less thrombogenic, easily manipulated, and provides a stable site for the venipuncture device.
- Puncture the vein quickly and efficiently to avoid excessive bruising.
- Remove the tourniquet promptly to prevent increased vascular pressure, which can cause bleeding through the vein wall around the infusion device.
- To stabilize the vein, stretch the skin proximal to the insertion site and anchor it firmly with your nondominant hand.

## What to consider

- Veins appear tortuous because of the skin's increased transparency and decreased elasticity.
- Veins appear large if venous pressure is adequate.
- Winged steel needles increase the risk of infiltration.
- Vein stabilization may be more difficult because of loose tissue.

## Managing complications of I.V. therapy

### Air embolism

What to look for
- Decreased blood pressure
- Increased central venous pressure
- Loss of consciousness
- Respiratory distress
- Unequal breath sounds
- Weak pulse

What causes it
- Empty solution container
- Secondary solution container emptied; air pushed down line by next container (primary)
- Disconnected tubing

What to do
- Discontinue the infusion.
- Place the patient in Trendelenburg's position to allow air to enter the right atrium and disperse through the pulmonary artery.
- Administer oxygen.
- Notify the doctor.
- Document the patient's condition and your interventions.

How to prevent it
- Purge the tubing of air completely before infusion.
- Use the air-detection device on the pump or the air-eliminating filter proximal to the I.V. site.
- Secure the connections.

# Allergic reaction

## What to look for

- Bronchospasm
- Itching
- Tearing eyes and runny nose
- Urticarial rash
- Wheezing
- Anaphylactic reaction occurring within minutes after exposure, including flushing, chills, anxiety, agitation, generalized itching, palpitations, paresthesia, throbbing in ears, wheezing, coughing, seizures, and cardiac arrest

## What causes it

- Allergens such as medications

## What to do

- If a reaction occurs, stop the infusion immediately.
- Maintain a patent airway.
- Notify the doctor.
- Administer an antihistaminic steroid, an anti-inflammatory, and antipyretic drugs, as ordered.
- Give aqueous epinephrine subcutaneously.
- Repeat the epinephrine dose at 3-minute intervals and as needed, or as ordered.
- Administer cortisone if ordered.

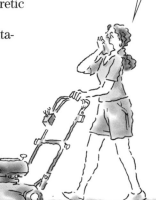

Allergies don't only sneak up on you when you mow the lawn! Watch your patients closely after administering a new drug.

## How to prevent it

- Obtain the patient's allergy history. Be aware of cross-allergies.
- Assist with test dosing.
- Monitor the patient carefully during the first 15 minutes of administering a new drug.

# Catheter dislodgment

## What to look for
- Catheter backed out of the vein
- Infusate infiltrating into tissue

## What causes it
- Loosened tape or tubing snagged in bedclothes, resulting in partial retraction of the catheter
- Dislodgment by a confused patient attempting to remove it

## What to do
- Remove the catheter.

## How to prevent it
- Tape the device securely on insertion.

# Circulatory overload

## What to look for

- Crackles
- Discomfort
- Increased blood pressure
- Large positive fluid balance (intake greater than output)
- Neck vein engorgement
- Respiratory distress

## What causes it

- Too rapid flow rate
- Miscalculation of fluid requirements
- Roller clamp loosened to allow run-on infusion

## What to do

- Raise the head of the bed.
- Administer oxygen as needed.
- Notify the doctor.
- Administer medications (usually furosemide) as ordered.

## How to prevent it

- Use a pump, controller, or rate minder for elderly or compromised patients.
- Recheck calculations of fluid requirements.
- Monitor the infusion frequently.

Watch the flow rate! Too much circulating fluid really puts me through the wringer!

# Hematoma

## What to look for
- Bruising around venipuncture site
- Tenderness at venipuncture site

## What causes it
- Leakage of blood into tissue
- Vein punctured through ventral wall at time of venipuncture

## What to do
- Remove the venipuncture device.
- Apply pressure and cold compresses to the affected area.
- Recheck for bleeding.
- Document the patient's condition and your interventions.

## How to prevent it
- Choose a vein that can accommodate the size of the intended venous access device.
- Release the tourniquet as soon as successful insertion is achieved.

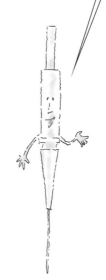

To prevent bruising, remember that size does matter...use the right-sized vein for the right-sized needle and catheter.

# Infiltration

## What to look for

- Blanching at site
- Continuing fluid infusion even when vein is occluded, although rate may decrease
- Cool skin around site
- Discomfort, burning, or pain at site
- Feeling of tightness at site
- Slower flow rate
- Swelling at and above I.V. site (may extend along entire limb)

## What causes it

- Device dislodged from vein or vein perforation

## What to do

- Remove the venipuncture device.
- Periodically assess circulation by checking for pulse and capillary refill.
- Restart the infusion in another limb.
- Notify the doctor.

## How to prevent it

- Check the I.V. site frequently, especially when using an I.V. pump.
- Don't obscure the area above the site with tape.
- Teach the patient to observe the I.V. site and report discomfort, pain, or swelling.

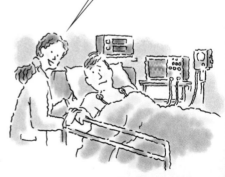

Make sure your patient knows to immediately report any discomfort, pain, or swelling at or around his I.V. site.

# Nerve, tendon, or ligament damage

## What to look for

- Delayed effects, including paralysis, numbness, and deformity
- Extreme pain (similar to electric shock when nerve is punctured)
- Numbness and muscle contraction

## What causes it

- Improper venipuncture technique, resulting in injury to surrounding nerves, tendons, or ligaments
- Taping too tight or improper splinting with arm board

## What to do

- Stop the procedure.
- Notify the doctor.

## How to prevent it

- Don't repeatedly penetrate tissues with the venipuncture device.
- Don't apply excessive pressure when taping or encircling the limb with tape.
- Pad the arm board and, if possible, pad the tape securing the arm board.

## Occlusion

### What to look for
- I.V. flow interrupted

### What causes it
- Blood backup in the line when the patient walks
- Hypercoagulable patient
- Intermittent device not flushed
- Line clamped too long

### What to do
- Use mild flush pressure during injection.
- Don't force the flush.
- If unsuccessful, reinsert the I.V. device.

### How to prevent it
- Maintain the I.V. flow rate.
- Flush promptly after intermittent piggyback administration.
- Have the patient walk with his arm folded to his chest to reduce the risk of blood backup.

# Phlebitis

## What to look for

- Redness at the tip of the catheter and along the vein
- Tenderness at the tip of the device and above
- Vein hard on palpation

## What causes it

- Clotting at the catheter tip (thrombophlebitis)
- Device left in the vein too long
- Friction from catheter movement in the vein
- Poor blood flow around the device
- Solution with high or low pH or high osmolarity

## What to do

- Remove the device.
- Apply a warm pack.
- Notify the doctor.
- Document the patient's condition and your interventions.

## How to prevent it

- Restart the infusion using a larger vein for initiating infusate, or restart with a smaller-gauge device to ensure adequate blood flow.
- Tape the device securely to prevent movement.

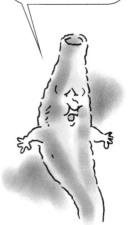

Suspect phlebitis if I become red, tender, and hard to the touch. Now, would you mind removing that device and bringing me a warm blanket?

## Severed catheter

### What to look for

- Leakage from the catheter shaft

### What causes it

- Catheter inadvertently cut by scissors
- Reinsertion of the needle into the catheter

### What to do

- If the broken portion of the catheter is visible, attempt to retrieve it. If unsuccessful, notify the doctor.
- If the broken portion of the catheter enters the bloodstream, place a tourniquet above the I.V. site to prevent its progression.
- Notify the doctor and the radiology department.
- Document the patient's condition and your interventions.

### How to prevent it

- Avoid using scissors around the I.V. site.
- Never reinsert the needle into the catheter.
- Remove the unsuccessfully inserted catheter and needle together.

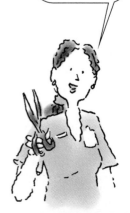

Just say no to having scissors around catheters!

# Systemic infection

## What to look for

- Contaminated I.V. site, usually with no visible signs of infection
- Fever, chills, and malaise for no apparent reason

## What causes it

- Failure to maintain aseptic technique during insertion or site care
- Immunocompromised patient
- Poor taping that permits the access device to move, which can introduce organisms into the bloodstream
- Prolonged indwelling time of device
- Severe phlebitis, which can set up ideal conditions for organism growth

## What to do

- Notify the doctor.
- Administer prescribed medications.
- Culture the site and the device.
- Monitor the patient's vital signs.

## How to prevent it

- Use meticulous aseptic technique when handling solutions and tubings, inserting the venipuncture device, and discontinuing the infusion.
- Secure all connections.
- Change I.V. solutions, tubing, and the access device at recommended times.

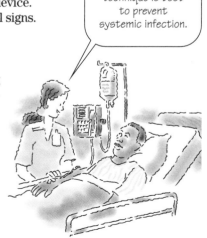

Aseptic technique is best to prevent systemic infection.

# Thrombophlebitis

## What to look for

- Reddened, swollen, and hardened vein
- Severe discomfort

## What causes it

- Thrombosis and inflammation

## What to do

- Remove the device; restart the infusion in the opposite limb if possible.
- Apply warm soaks.
- Watch for I.V. therapy-related infection. (Thrombi provide an excellent environment for bacterial growth.)
- Notify the doctor.

## How to prevent it

- Check the site frequently.
- Remove the device at the first sign of redness and tenderness.

# Thrombosis

## What to look for

- Painful, reddened, and swollen vein
- Sluggish or stopped I.V. flow

## What causes it

- Injury to the endothelial cells of the vein wall, allowing platelets to adhere and thrombus to form

## What to do

- Remove the device; restart the infusion in the opposite limb if possible.
- Apply warm soaks.
- Watch for I.V. therapy-related infection. (Thrombi provide an excellent environment for bacterial growth.)
- Notify the doctor.

## How to prevent it

- Use proper venipuncture technique to reduce injury to the vein.

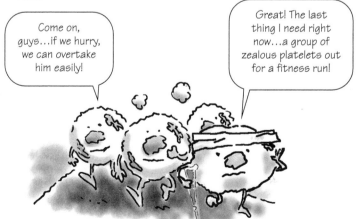

# Vein irritation at the I.V. site

## What to look for
- Pain during infusion
- Possible blanching if vasospasm occurs
- Rapidly developing signs of phlebitis
- Red skin over the vein during infusion

## What causes it
- Solution with a high or low pH or high osmolarity, such as 40 mEq/L of potassium chloride, phenytoin, and some antibiotics, such as vancomycin and nafcillin

## What to do
- Slow the flow rate.
- Try using an electronic flow device to achieve a steady, regulated flow.

## How to prevent it
- Dilute solutions before administration. For example, give antibiotics in a 250-ml solution rather than a 100-ml solution.
- If the drug has a low pH, ask a pharmacist if it can be buffered with sodium bicarbonate. (Refer to facility policy.)
- If long-term therapy of an irritating drug is planned, ask the doctor to use a central I.V. line.

# Venous spasm

## What to look for
- Blanched skin over the vein
- Pain along the vein
- Sluggish flow rate when the clamp is completely open

## What causes it
- Administration of cold fluids or blood
- Severe vein irritation from irritating drugs or fluids
- Very rapid flow rate (with fluids at room temperature)

## What to do
- Apply warm soaks over the vein and surrounding area.
- Slow the flow rate.

## How to prevent it
- Use a blood warmer for blood or packed red blood cells when appropriate.

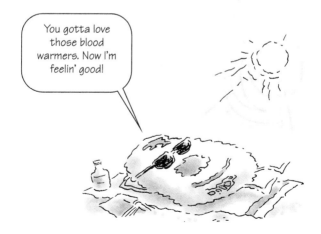

# Central venous therapy

# 3

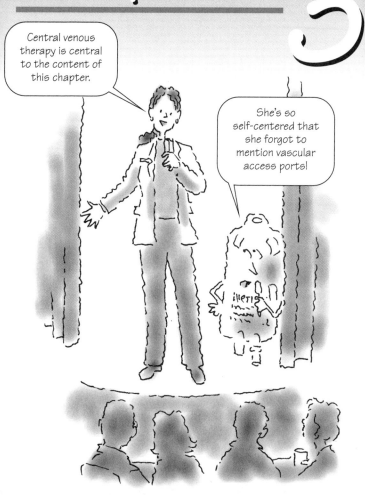

# Understanding CV therapy

## CV therapy basics

### Why it's done

- To access central venous (CV) system in an emergency
- To infuse a large volume of fluid
- To administer multiple infusions
- To administer long-term venous therapy

### The pros

- Provides access to the central veins
- Allows for rapid infusion of medications or large amounts of fluids
- Provides a way to draw blood samples and measure CV pressure (CVP), an important indicator of circulatory function
- Reduces the need for repeated venipunctures, which decreases the patient's anxiety and preserves (or restores) the peripheral veins
- Reduces the risk of vein irritation from infusing irritating or caustic substances

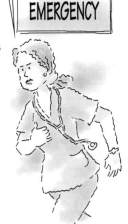

CV therapy is the order when there's an emergency.

EMERGENCY

### The cons

- Requires more time and skill to insert than a peripheral I.V. catheter
- Costs more to maintain than a peripheral I.V. catheter
- Carries a risk of life-threatening complications, such as air embolism, perforation of the vessel and adjacent organs, pneumothorax, sepsis, and thrombus formation

## Comparing CV catheter types

## Peripherally inserted central catheter

Key facts

- Also called *long-line catheter*
- Made of silicone or polyurethane
- Inserted through a peripheral vein, with the tip ending in the superior vena cava
- Commonly used in women who require I.V. therapy because of severe morning sickness and in patients with recurrent infections, acquired immunodeficiency syndrome (AIDS), cancer, and sickle cell anemia

> Wouldn't want to be caught hanging without my trusty PICC on these long treks over CV terrain.

**Memory jogger**

Here's the long and short of it! The other name for peripherally inserted catheters will help you remember why they're used: Long-line catheters are for long-term use.

## Why it's used

- To transfuse blood
- To infuse caustic drugs or solutions
- To administer CV therapy for 5 days to several months
- To enable repeated venous access

## The pros

- Provides long-term access to central veins (may be left in place for up to 1 year)
- Especially useful if a patient doesn't have reliable routes for short-term I.V. therapy
- Can be used to administer analgesics (including opioids), antibiotics, blood products, chemotherapy, immunoglobulins, and total parenteral nutrition (TPN)
- May prevent such complications as pneumothorax, which may occur with a CV line
- Antithrombogenic properties minimize the risk of blood clots and phlebitis
- Available in single- or double-lumen configurations and with or without guide wires
- Extremely cost-effective compared to other long-term and short-term CV catheters

## The cons

- May not be suitable for patients with bruises, scarring, or sclerosis from earlier multiple venipunctures at the intended peripherally inserted central catheter (PICC) site; considered a last resort for these patients
- When used to administer a medication or flush the catheter, tuberculin or 3-ml syringes with a PICC create too much pressure (pounds per square inch) in the line, which can cause the device to burst

# Tunneled catheter

## Key facts
- Designed for long-term use
- Styles include Broviac, Hickman, and Groshong catheters; available in single-, double-, triple-, or multilumen configurations
- Vary in size

## Why it's used
- To treat patients who have poor peripheral venous access or who need long-term daily infusions, such as those with AIDS, anemia, bone or organ infections, cancer, intestinal malabsorption, and other chronic diseases
- To administer antibiotics, blood products, chemotherapy, and TPN

## The pros
- Radiopaque (placement can be checked by X-ray)
- Usually made of silicone; much less likely to cause thrombosis than catheters made of polyurethane or polyvinyl chloride
- Minimal irritation or damage to the vein lining
- Cuffs encourage tissue growth at the exit site and keep bacteria out of venous circulation

The trick to maneuvering through these tunnel catheters is to stay low and hope your headlamp batteries hold out!

## The cons
- Better suited for home care because they're designed for long-term use

# Nontunneled catheter

## Key facts
- Also called *central catheter*

## Why it's used
- To briefly continue I.V. therapy after hospitalization

## The pros
- Useful in an emergency because of easy insertion (not tunneled under skin)
- Radiopaque (placement can be checked by X-ray)
- May be impregnated with heparin, chlorhexidine, or an antibiotic

## The cons
- May be easily dislodged by patient movement
- May be more thrombogenic than tunneled catheters
- May be associated with a higher risk of infection than tunneled catheters
- Designed for short-term use

## Comparing CV catheter configurations

## Short-term, single-lumen catheter

Key facts
- Polyurethane or silicone rubber (Silastic)
- Approximately 8″ (20.3 cm) long
- Variety of lumen gauges

Why it's used
- To provide short-term CV access
- To provide emergency access to the CV system
- To enable infusion when a patient requires only a single lumen

*Picture this!*

### A single lumen for a quick fix

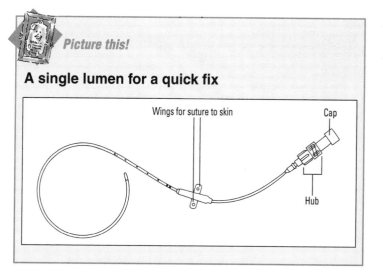

Wings for suture to skin    Cap

Hub

## The pros

- Can be inserted at the bedside
- Easily removed
- Stiffness aids CV pressure monitoring

## The cons

- Limited functionality
- Should be changed every 3 to 7 days (depending on your facility's policy)

## What to do

- Minimize patient motion and activities.
- Assess frequently for signs of infection and clot formation.

# Short-term, multilumen catheter

## Key facts

- Polyurethane or silicone rubber (Silastic)
- Double, triple, or quadruple lumen at $\frac{3}{4}''$ (1.9-cm) intervals
- Variety of lumen gauges

## Why it's used

- To provide short-term CV access
- To administer multiple infusions in patients with limited insertion sites

## The pros

- Can be inserted at bedside
- Easily removed
- Stiffness aids CV pressure monitoring
- Allows infusion of multiple solutions through the same catheter

*Picture this!*

## Multiple lumens for many infusions

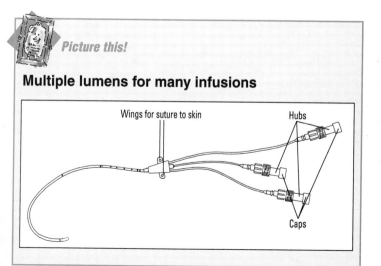

Wings for suture to skin

Hubs

Caps

## The cons

- Limited functionality
- Needs to be changed every 3 to 7 days

## What to do

- Know the gauge and purpose of each lumen.
- Use the same lumen for the same task (for example, to administer TPN or to collect a blood sample).

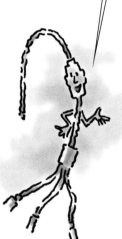

I'm a multi-tasker — a product of my time!

# Broviac catheter

## Key facts

- Silicone rubber (Silastic)
- Approximately 35″ (88.9 cm) long
- Open end with clamp
- Dacron cuff 11¾″ (29.9 cm) from hub
- Identical to Hickman catheter except smaller inner lumen

## Why it's used

- To provide long-term CV access
- To administer infusions to a patient with small central vessels (pediatric and elderly patients)

## The pros

- Smaller lumen than other CV catheters (provides greater comfort)

**Picture this!**

**Broviac catheter: A long-term solution for small central vessels**

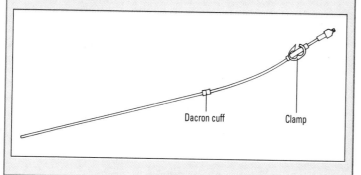

Dacron cuff          Clamp

## The cons
- Small lumen may limit uses
- Doesn't allow simultaneous infusion of multiple solutions

## What to do
- Check your facility's policy before drawing or administering blood products.
- Flush the catheter daily when not in use with 3 to 5 ml of heparin (10 units/ml) and before and after each medication administration, using the SASH (saline, administer, saline, heparin) protocol.

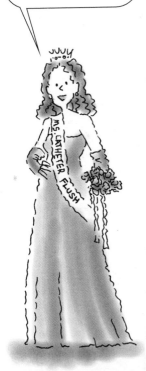

I'd like to thank the SASH protocol for making me the catheter flusher I am today!

# Groshong catheter

## Key facts

- Tunneled catheter
- Silicone rubber (Silastic)
- Approximately 35″ (88.9 cm) long
- Closed end with pressure-sensitive, two-way valve
- Dacron cuff
- Available with single or double lumen

## Why it's used

- To provide long-term CV access
- To administer infusions to a patient with heparin allergy

*Picture this!*

### Groshong catheter: When heparin is needed

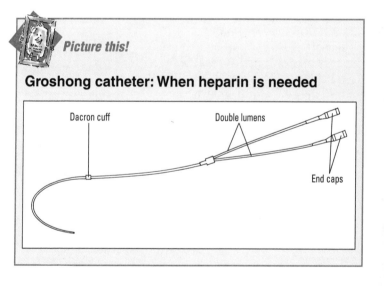

Dacron cuff     Double lumens

End caps

## The pros

- Less thrombogenic than catheters made with polyvinyl chloride
- Pressure sensitive, two-way valve (eliminates heparin flushes)
- Dacron cuff anchors catheter and prevents bacterial migration

## The cons

- Requires surgical insertion
- Tears and kinks easily
- Blunt end makes it difficult to clear substances from tip

## What to do

- Apply dressings to the two surgical sites after insertion.
- Handle the catheter gently.
- Check the external portion frequently for kinks or leaks. (A repair kit is available.)
- Flush the lumen with enough saline solution to clear the catheter, especially after drawing or administering blood.
- Change the end caps weekly.

# Hickman catheter

## Key facts
- Tunneled catheter
- Silicone rubber (Silastic)
- Approximately 35″ (88.9 cm) long
- Open end with clamp
- Dacron cuff 11¾″ (29.9 cm) from hub

## Why it's used
- To enable at-home therapy
- To provide long-term CV access

## The pros
- Dacron cuff prevents excess motion and organism migration
- Clamps eliminate need for Valsalva's maneuver

*Picture this!*

**Hickman catheter: Ideal for at-home therapy**

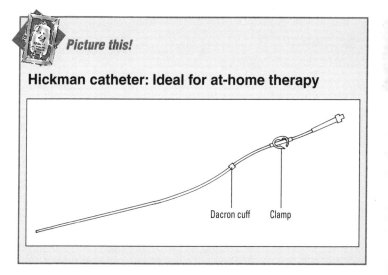

Dacron cuff      Clamp

## The cons

- Requires surgical insertion
- Has an open end
- Requires a doctor for removal
- Tears and kinks easily

## What to do

- Apply dressings to the two surgical sites after insertion.
- Handle the catheter gently.
- Observe frequently for kinks or tears. (A repair kit is available.)
- Clamp the catheter whenever it becomes disconnected or open, using a nonserrated clamp.
- Flush the catheter daily when not in use with 3 to 5 ml of heparin (10 units/ml) and before and after each medication administration, using the SASH protocol.

# Hickman-Broviac catheter

### Key facts
- Hickman and Broviac catheters combined into one catheter

### Why it's used
- To provide long-term CV access
- To administer multiple infusions

### The pros
- Double-lumen Hickman catheter allows blood sampling and administration
- Broviac lumen delivers I.V. fluids, including TPN

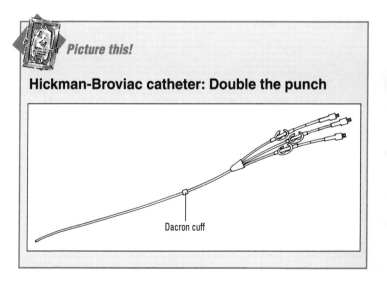

*Picture this!*

**Hickman-Broviac catheter: Double the punch**

Dacron cuff

## The cons

- Requires surgical insertion
- Has an open end
- Requires a doctor for removal
- Tears and kinks easily

## What to do

- Know the purpose and function of each lumen.
- Label the lumens to prevent confusion.
- Change the end caps weekly.
- Flush the catheter daily when not in use with 3 to 5 ml of heparin (10 units/ml) and before and after each medication administration, using the SASH protocol.

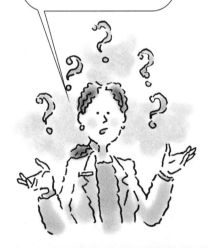

Not knowing the purpose and function of each lumen isn't an option. Clearly label all lumens to avoid confusion and costly mistakes.

# Long-line catheter

## Key facts

- PICC
- Silicone rubber (Silastic)
- 20″ to 24″ (51 to 61 cm) long
- Available in 14G, 16G, 18G, 20G, and 22G

## Why it's used

- To provide long-term CV access
- To administer infusions to a patient with poor central access
- To administer infusions to a patient at risk for fatal complications from insertion at central access sites
- To administer infusions to a patient who needs CV access or has had or will have head and neck surgery

**Picture this!**

### Peripherally inserted long-line catheter

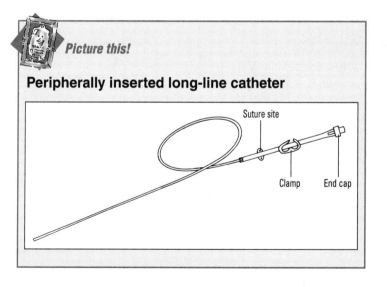

Suture site

Clamp

End cap

## The pros

- Peripherally inserted
- Can be inserted at the bedside with minimal complications
- May be inserted by a trained, skilled, competent registered nurse in most states
- Single lumen or double lumen available

## The cons

- May occlude smaller peripheral vessels
- May alter CV pressure measurements

## What to do

- Insert the catheter above the antecubital fossa.
- Check the insertion site frequently for signs of phlebitis and thrombus formation.
- Use an arm board if necessary; it may be hard to keep the catheter immobile.

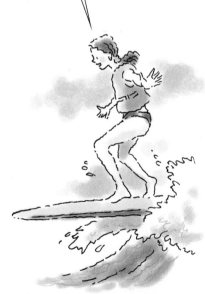

I can picture the headline for my next article in *Surfer Magazine*: "Nurse hangs 10 on one extreme arm board for a VERY long-line catheter!"

## Preparing for CV therapy

## Selecting the insertion site

### What to consider

- Type of catheter
- Patient's anatomy and age
- Duration of therapy
- Vessel integrity and accessibility
- History of previous chest surgery (such as mastectomy)
- Presence of chest trauma
- Possible complications

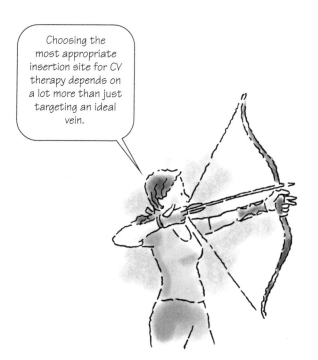

Choosing the most appropriate insertion site for CV therapy depends on a lot more than just targeting an ideal vein.

# Cephalic and basilic veins

## The pros

- Least risk of major complications among all CV catheters
- Easy to keep dressing in place

## The cons

- Possible cutdown required
- Possible difficulty locating antecubital fossa in obese patients
- Hard to keep elbow immobile, especially in children

*Picture this!*

## Veins used in CV therapy

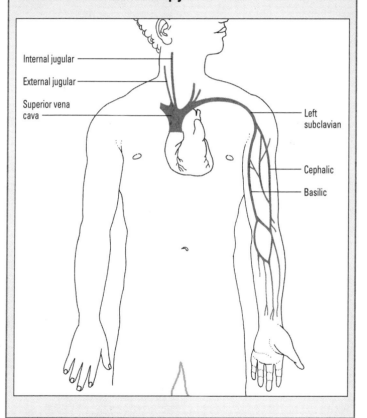

Internal jugular

External jugular

Superior vena cava

Left subclavian

Cephalic

Basilic

# External jugular vein

## The pros

- Easy access, especially in children
- Decreased risk of pneumothorax and arterial puncture

## The cons

- Less direct route
- Lower flow rate (increases risk of thrombus)
- Hard to keep dressing in place
- Tortuous vein, especially in elderly patients

# Internal jugular vein

## The pros
- Short, direct route to the right atrium
- Catheter stability, resulting in less movement with respiration
- Decreased risk of pneumothorax

## The cons
- Proximity to the common carotid artery (If the artery is punctured during catheter insertion, uncontrolled hemorrhage, emboli, or impedance to flow can result.)
- Hard to keep dressing in place
- Proximity to the trachea

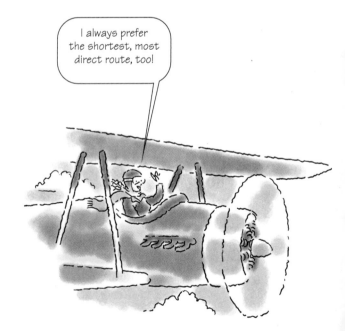

# Subclavian vein

## The pros
- Easy access
- Easy to keep dressing in place
- High flow rate (reduces risk of thrombus)

## The cons
- Proximity to the subclavian artery (If the artery is punctured during catheter insertion, hemorrhage can occur.)
- Hard to control bleeding
- Increased risk of pneumothorax

## Maintaining CV infusions

## Monitoring a patient with a CV catheter

*What to do*

- Tailor your assessment and interventions to the particular catheter insertion site.
- Closely monitor the patient's respiratory status, watching for dyspnea, shortness of breath, and sudden chest pain if the catheter insertion site is close to major thoracic organs (as with a subclavian or internal jugular site).
- Monitor the catheter's position carefully. A poorly positioned catheter, especially one inserted into the internal or external jugular veins, can cause kinking, can make dressing changes difficult, and can make it impossible to maintain an occlusive dressing.
- Monitor the patient's cardiac status.
- Be aware that catheter insertion can cause arrhythmias if the catheter enters the right ventricle and irritates the cardiac muscle.
- Make sure a chest X-ray is ordered to confirm the location of the catheter tip in the superior vena cava before starting infusions.

> Tailor how you monitor and intervene according to the catheter site.

- To begin the infusion, connect the I.V. tubing or intermittent cap to the catheter hub.
- If the line is to be used for infusion, run an isotonic fluid at a rate no greater than 20 ml/hour until catheter placement is confirmed.
- After the X-ray confirmation, adjust the flow rate as prescribed.
- Obtain a blood return of 3 to 5 ml of free-flowing blood from the catheter before each use.

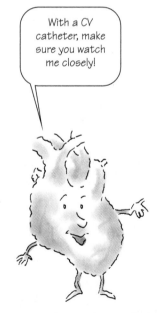

# Applying a CV catheter dressing

## What to do

- Maintain sterile technique.
- Place a sterile dressing over the insertion site of a short-term catheter or the exit site of a peripherally inserted central or tunneled catheter.
- Clean the site with chlorhexidine solution.
- Cover the site with a transparent, semipermeable dressing.
- Seal the dressing with nonporous tape, checking that all edges are well secured.
- Label the dressing with the date and time, your initials, and the catheter length.
- Place the patient in a comfortable position, and re-assess his status.
- Elevate the head of the bed 45 degrees to help the patient breathe more easily.
- Keep the site clean and dry to prevent infection.
- Keep the dressing occlusive to prevent air embolism and contamination.

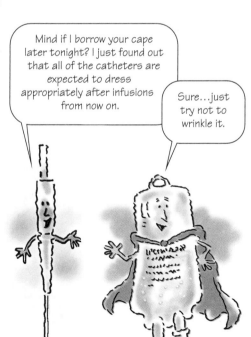

Mind if I borrow your cape later tonight? I just found out that all of the catheters are expected to dress appropriately after infusions from now on.

Sure...just try not to wrinkle it.

# Changing a CV catheter dressing

## What to do

- Gather the necessary equipment.
- Wash your hands.
- Place the patient in a comfortable position.
- Prepare a sterile field.

*Help desk*

### Changing a CV dressing

After you assemble all needed equipment:

**Remove the old dressing.**

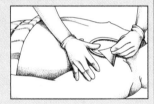

**Clean the insertion site.**

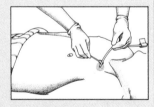

**Re-dress the site.**

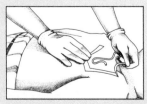

- Open the bag, placing it outside the sterile field but still within reach.

## Removing the old dressing
- Put on clean gloves and remove the old dressing.
- Inspect the dressing for signs of infection.
- Culture discharge at the site or on the old dressing.
- Discard the dressing and gloves.
- Check the insertion site for signs of infiltration or infection, such as redness, swelling, tenderness, or drainage.
- Report an infection to the doctor immediately, and document your findings.
- Check the position of the catheter.

## Cleaning the insertion site
- Put on sterile gloves.
- Clean the skin around the catheter with chlorhexidine, wiping outward from the insertion site in a back-and-forth or side-to-side motion.
- Don't use solutions containing acetone to clean the skin around the site; they may cause some catheters to disintegrate.

## Re-dressing the site
- Re-dress the site with a transparent semipermeable dressing.
- If the catheter is taped (not sutured) to the skin, carefully replace the soiled tape with sterile tape, using the chevron method.
- Label the dressing with the date, the time, and your initials.
- Discard all used items properly; reposition the patient comfortably.

# Flushing a CV catheter

## What to do

- Select a flushing solution
  – Heparinized saline solution is available in premixed, 10-ml multidose vials, in concentrations from 10 units of heparin/ml to 100 units of heparin/ml.
  – Saline solution is preferred by some facilities because heparin isn't always necessary to keep the line open.
- Flush the CV catheter with heparin solution routinely (according to your facility's policy) to maintain patency. Two-way valve catheters, such as the Groshong catheter, require only saline flushes to maintain patency.
- Never force the flush solution into a catheter if you meet resistance.
- Obtain a return of 3 to 5 ml of free-flowing blood from the catheter before each use.
- Determine the number of flushes per day; recommendations range from once every 8 hours to once per day.
- Clean the cap with an alcohol swab (using a 70% alcohol solution).
- Allow the cap to dry.
- Inject the recommended or prescribed type and amount of flushing solution.

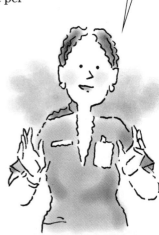

It's recommended that you flush CV catheters as frequently as once every 8 hours.

- Prevent blood backflow and possible clotting in the line by:
  – keeping your thumb on the plunger of the syringe to maintain positive pressure
  – engaging the clamping mechanism in the central line
  – withdrawing the syringe.

## What to consider

- Use the lowest possible effective heparin concentration (higher concentrations can interfere with the patient's clotting factors).
- Amount of flushing solution:
  – Infusion Nurses Society: At least twice the volume capacity of the catheter and add-on devices
  – Facility policies: 3 to 5 ml of solution commonly accepted, but not universal; some policies allow for as much as 10 ml of solution
- When giving incompatible medications, flush the catheter with heparin or normal saline solution before and after administration.
- When using a CV catheter with a two-way valve, flush the catheter with saline solution once per day when not in use.
- When using multilumen catheters, all lumens (unless it's a valved catheter) should be flushed regularly with heparin or saline solution, depending on your facility's policy and practice.

# Changing CV catheter tubing

## What to do

- Explain to the patient what will be done.
- Wash your hands.
- Place a 2 × 2 sterile gauze pad under the needle or catheter hub to create a sterile field.
- Reduce the I.V. flow rate.
- Remove the old spike and tubing from the bag.
- Keeping the old spike in an upright position above the patient's heart, insert the new spike into the I.V. container.
- Prime the system.
- Instruct the patient to perform Valsalva's maneuver.
- Quickly disconnect the old tubing from the needle or catheter hub, being careful not to dislodge the venipuncture device.
- If it's difficult to disconnect, use a hemostat to hold the hub securely while the end of the tubing is twisted and removed.

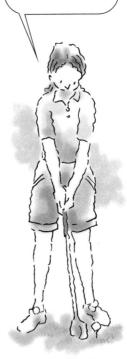

Just like with golf shoes, sometimes you've got to remove your old spikes and insert new ones!

# Drawing blood from a CV catheter with an evacuated tube

## What to do

- Identify the patient using two identifiers (not the patient's room number).
- Wash your hands.
- Put on sterile gloves.
- Stop the I.V. infusion.
- Place an injection cap on the lumen of the catheter.
- If multiple infusions are running, stop them and wait 1 minute before drawing blood from the catheter.
- Clean the end of the injection cap with antiseptic swabs (povidone-iodine and alcohol).
- Place a 5-ml lavender-top evacuated tube into its plastic sleeve. Use this tube to collect and discard the filling volume of the catheter, plus an extra 2 to 3 ml. (Most studies indicate that about 5 ml is enough blood to discard.)
- Check your facility's protocol. At some facilities the first 5 ml of blood isn't discarded if the patient is scheduled for multiple blood studies; the blood is instead infused back into the patient after the sample is drawn.
- Insert the needleless device into the injection cap of the catheter.

> Be sure to check your facility's policy about the types of tubes you need and the amount of blood you should discard before drawing blood from a CV catheter.

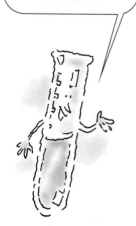

- When blood stops flowing into the tube, remove and discard the tube, if appropriate.
- Put the blood in the appropriate evacuated tubes for the ordered blood tests; label the tubes, and send them to the laboratory.
- Flush the catheter with saline solution and resume the infusion.
- Heparinize the catheter if you aren't going to use the lumen immediately.
- Ask the patient to raise his arms over his head, turn on his side, cough, or perform Valsalva's maneuver if you can't get blood flowing from the catheter (the tip of the catheter could be against the vessel wall). You may also try flushing the catheter with saline solution before making another attempt to draw blood.

# Drawing blood from a CV catheter with a syringe

What to do

- Identify the patient using two identifiers (not the patient's room number).
- Stop all infusions.
- Select the port from which to withdraw the blood (preferably a 16G or 18G; no smaller than a 20G).
- Put on sterile gloves.
- Disconnect the tubing or saline lock cap, using sterile technique.
- If the catheter has a clamp, use it before disconnecting; if the catheter doesn't have a clamp, have the patient perform Valsalva's maneuver.
- Insert the syringe and withdraw 5 ml of blood.
- Discard the syringe.
- Connect a second syringe.
- Draw the amount of blood you need.
- Flush the catheter with the recommended amount of saline solution or heparin. (The amount depends on the type of catheter and the frequency and type of infusions. Check the manufacturer's recommendations and your facility's policy.)
- Place the blood in the evacuated tubes, label the tubes, and send them to the laboratory.

> After the tubes are labeled, they can be sent off to the lab!

# Removing a CV catheter

## What to do

- Explain to the patient what will be done.
- Wash your hands.
- Place the patient in a supine position to prevent emboli.
- Put on clean gloves.
- Turn off all infusions and prepare a sterile field.
- Remove the old dressing.
- Put on sterile gloves.
- Prepare the site with alcohol.
- Inspect the site for signs of drainage or inflammation.
- Clip the sutures and remove the catheter in a slow, even motion while the patient performs Valsalva's maneuver (to prevent air emboli).
- Seal the insertion site by applying povidone-iodine ointment.
- Inspect the catheter to see if any portions have broken off during the removal. If this has occurred, notify the doctor immediately and monitor the patient closely for signs of distress.
- If a culture is needed, clip approximately 1″ (2.5 cm) off the distal end of the catheter, letting it drop into the sterile specimen container.
- Place a transparent, semipermeable dressing over the site.

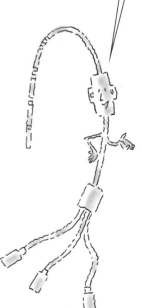

- Label the dressing with the date, time, and your initials.
- Properly dispose of the I.V. tubing and equipment you used.
- Check for signs of respiratory decompensation, possibly indicating air emboli.
- Check for signs of bleeding, such as blood on the dressing, decreased blood pressure, increased heart rate, paleness, or diaphoresis.
- Document the time and date of the catheter removal.
- Document any complications, such as catheter shearing, bleeding, and respiratory distress. Record signs of blood or drainage as well as redness or swelling of the site.

## What to consider

- Insidious bleeding may develop after removing the catheter. Remember that some vessels, such as the subclavian vein, aren't easily compressed. Even if the site remains sealed and the risk of air emboli has passed (generally 72 hours after removal of the catheter), you may still need to apply a dry dressing to the site.

## Managing common problems in CV therapy

### Disconnected catheter

What causes it

- Catheter not securely connected to tubing
- Patient movement

What to do

- Apply a catheter clamp if available.
- Place a sterile syringe or catheter plug in the catheter hub.
- Change the I.V. extension set; don't reconnect the contaminated tubing.
- Clean the catheter hub with alcohol or povidone-iodine solution; don't soak the hub.
- Connect clean I.V. tubing or a heparin lock plug to the site.
- Restart the infusion.

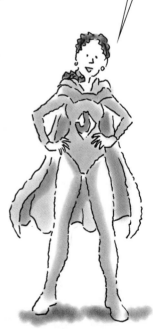

Disconnected catheters and leaky sites, beware! CV troubleshooting is my specialty!

# Fluid leaking at insertion site

## What causes it
- Displaced catheter
- Fibrin sheath
- Lymph fluid leaking from tract
- Tear in catheter

## What to do
- Check the patient for signs of distress.
- Change the dressing and observe the site for redness.
- Notify the doctor.
- Obtain an X-ray order.
- Prepare for a catheter change if necessary.
- Use a repair kit if a tear occurs in a Hickman, Groshong, or Broviac catheter.

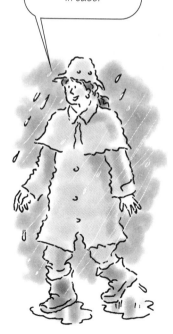

# Fluid won't infuse

## What causes it

- Closed clamp
- Displaced or kinked catheter
- Thrombus

## What to do

- Check the infusion system for kinks, and make sure the clamps aren't too tight.
- Change the patient's position.
- Remove the dressing and examine the external portion of the catheter.
- If a kink isn't apparent, obtain an X-ray order.
- Try to withdraw blood.
- Try a gentle flush with saline solution. (The doctor may order a thrombolytic flush.)

# Unable to draw blood

## What causes it
- Catheter movement against vessel wall with negative pressure
- Closed clamp
- Thrombus

## What to do
- Check the infusion system and clamps.
- Change the patient's position.
- Remove the dressing, and examine the external portion of the catheter.
- Obtain an X-ray order to confirm placement.

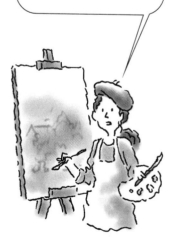

Can't draw blood? Check for kinks in the infusion system, change the patient's position, and check the catheter for proper placement.

# Managing complications of CV therapy

## Air embolism

### What to look for

- Change in or loss of consciousness
- Churning murmur over precordium
- Decreased blood pressure
- Increased CVP
- Respiratory distress
- Unequal breath sounds
- Weak pulse

### What causes it

- Intake of air into the CV system during catheter insertion or tubing changes
- Inadvertent opening, cutting, or breaking of the catheter

### What to do

- Clamp the catheter immediately.
- Reassure the patient.
- Turn the patient on his left side, with his head down, so air can enter the right atrium, preventing it from entering the pulmonary artery.
- Administer oxygen.
- Notify the doctor.
- Document your interventions.
- Don't have the patient perform Valsalva's maneuver because a large intake of air would worsen the situation.

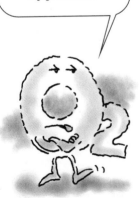

I can tell when I'm not wanted...Now, who do I see if want to air my grievances?

## How to prevent it

- Purge all air from the tubing before hookup.
- Teach the patient to perform Valsalva's maneuver during catheter insertion and tubing changes.
- Use an infusion-control device with air-detection capability.
- Use luer-lock tubing or tape connections, or use locking devices for all connections.

# Chylothorax, hemothorax, hydrothorax, or pneumothorax

## What to look for

- Abnormal chest X-ray
- Chest pain
- Cyanosis
- Decreased breath sounds on affected side
- Dyspnea
- Decreased hemoglobin level because of blood pooling (with hemothorax)

## What causes it

- Lung puncture caused by catheter during insertion or exchange over a guide wire
- Large blood vessel puncture with bleeding inside or outside the lung
- Lymph node puncture with leakage of lymph fluid
- Infusion of solution into the chest area through the catheter

## What to do

- Stop the infusion.
- Notify the doctor.
- Reassure the patient.
- Remove the catheter or assist with its removal.
- Administer prescribed oxygen.

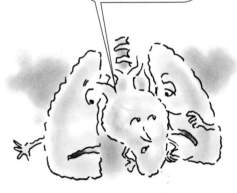

- Set up and assist with chest tube insertion.
- Document your interventions.

## How to prevent it

- Position the patient with his head down with a towel roll between the scapulae to dilate and expose the internal jugular or subclavian vein as much as possible during catheter insertion.
- Assess for early signs of fluid infiltration such as swelling in shoulder, neck, chest, or arm area.
- Ensure patient immobilization with adequate preparation before the procedure and adequate restraint during the procedure; active patients may need to be sedated or taken to the operating room for CV catheter insertion.
- Minimize patient activity after insertion, especially if a peripheral CV catheter is used.

# Local infection

## What to look for

- Fever, chills, malaise
- Local rash or pustules
- Exudate of purulent material
- Redness, warmth, tenderness, and swelling at insertion or exit site

## What causes it

- Failure to maintain sterile technique during catheter insertion or care
- Failure to comply with dressing change protocol
- Wet or soiled dressing left on site
- Immunosuppression
- Irritated suture line

## What to do

- Monitor the patient's temperature frequently.
- Culture the site if there's drainage.
- Re-dress the site aseptically.
- Use antibiotic ointment locally if ordered.
- Treat systemically with antibiotics or antifungals, depending on culture results and the doctor's order.
- Remove the catheter if ordered.
- Document your interventions.

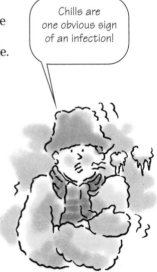

Chills are one obvious sign of an infection!

## How to prevent it

- Maintain strict sterile technique.
- Adhere to dressing change protocols.
- Teach the patient about restrictions on swimming and bathing. (Patients with adequate white blood cell counts may swim and bathe if the doctor allows.)
- Change a wet or soiled dressing immediately.
- Change the dressing more frequently if the catheter is located in a femoral area or near a tracheostomy.
- Do catheter care first, then complete tracheostomy care.

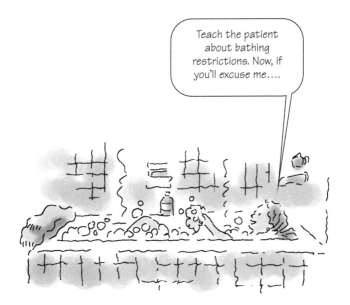

## Systemic infection

### What to look for

- Elevated urine glucose level
- Fever and chills without other apparent reason
- Leukocytosis
- Malaise
- Nausea and vomiting

### What causes it

- Contaminated catheter or infusate
- Failure to maintain sterile technique during solution hookup
- Frequent opening of catheter or long-term use of single I.V. access
- Immunosuppression

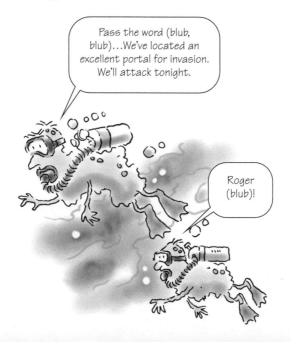

## What to do

- Draw central and peripheral blood cultures; if the same organism is present in both, the catheter is the primary source of sepsis and should be removed. If cultures don't match but are positive, the catheter may be removed or the infection may be treated through the catheter.
- Treat the patient with the prescribed antibiotic regimen.
- Culture the tip of the catheter if removed.
- Assess for other sources of infection.
- Monitor vital signs closely.
- Document your interventions.

## How to prevent it

- Examine infusate for cloudiness and turbidity before infusing.
- Check the fluid container for leaks.
- Monitor urine glucose level in patients receiving TPN; if greater than 2+, suspect early sepsis.
- Use strict sterile technique for hookup and disconnection of fluids.
- Change the catheter frequently to decrease the risk of infection.
- Keep the system closed as much as possible.
- Teach the patient sterile technique.

# Thrombosis

## What to look for

- Edema at the puncture site
- Fever and malaise
- Ipsilateral swelling of the arm, neck, and face
- Pain
- Tachycardia

## What causes it

- Improper catheter tip location in the subclavian or brachio-cephalic vein
- Sluggish flow rate
- Patient's hematopoietic status
- Repeated or long-term use of the same vein
- Preexisting cardiovascular disease
- Vein irritation during insertion

## What to do

- Stop the infusion.
- Notify the doctor.
- Infuse anticoagulant doses of heparin if ordered.
- Verify thrombosis with diagnostic studies as ordered.
- Don't use the limb on the affected side for subsequent venipuncture.
- Document your interventions.

## How to prevent it

- Maintain flow through the catheter at a steady rate with an infusion pump, or flush at regular intervals.
- Verify that the catheter tip is in the superior vena cava before using the catheter.

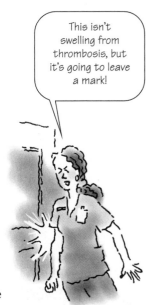

# Understanding VAP implantation and infusion

## VAP basics

### Key facts

- Indwelling catheter attached to a vascular access port (VAP) is surgically tunneled under the skin until the catheter tip lies in the superior vena cava

### Why it's used

- To access the CV system when a peripheral catheter isn't suitable
- To enable epidural, intra-arterial, or intraperitoneal placement

### The pros

- Function much like long-term CV catheters
- No external parts
- Minimal activity restrictions
- Few self-care measures for the patient to learn and perform
- Few dressing changes (except when accessed and used to maintain continuous infusions or intermittent infusion devices)

### The cons

- May be more difficult for the patient to manage than other catheters
- Accessing requires insertion of a specialized needle through subcutaneous tissue.

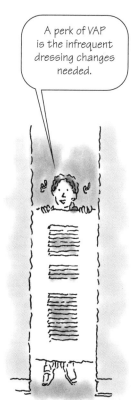

A perk of VAP is the infrequent dressing changes needed.

*Picture this!*

## Understanding implantable pumps

An implantable pump is usually placed in a subcutaneous pocket made in the abdomen below the umbilicus. It has two chambers separated by a bellows. One chamber contains the I.V. solution and the other contains a charging fluid. The charging fluid chamber exerts continuous pressure on the bellows, forcing the infusion solution through the silicone outlet catheter into a central vein. The pump also has an auxiliary septum that can be used to deliver bolus injections of medication. Generally, the pump is indicated for patients who require continuous, low-volume infusions.

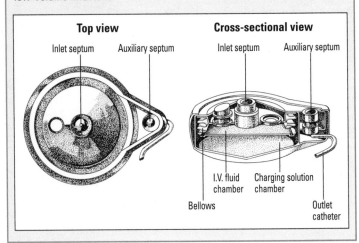

**Top view**

Inlet septum     Auxiliary septum

**Cross-sectional view**

Inlet septum     Auxiliary septum

I.V. fluid     Charging solution
chamber        chamber

Bellows

Outlet
catheter

- Accessing may be uncomfortable for patients who fear or dislike needles.
- Implantation and removal requires surgery and possible hospitalization.

## Performing a VAP infusion

## Selecting a VAP needle

What to consider

- Use only noncoring needles with a VAP.
- Needle gauge
  - 19G needle—for blood infusion or withdrawal
  - 20G needle—for most infusions other than blood infusion or withdrawal, including TPN
  - 22G needle—for flushing
- Needle type
  - A right-angle, noncoring needle is most commonly used.
  - Rarely, a longer needle, such as a straight, 2-inch noncoring needle, is used to access a deeply implanted port.
  - A straight or right-angle needle is used to inject a bolus into a top-entry port.
  - A straight, noncoring needle is used only for side-entry ports.
  - Right-angle needles are preferred for continuous infusions (easier to secure to the patient).

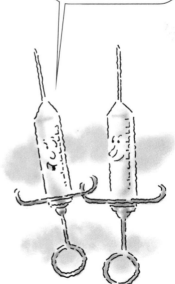

I guess we aren't the only sharp ones around here...those nurses need to know all the angles, too!

## Accessing a top-entry VAP

### What to do

- Numb the area with a topical anesthetic cream, ice, or ethyl chloride spray, depending on the doctor's order or your facility's policy.
- Assemble the equipment.
- Palpate the area over the port to locate the port septum.
- Anchor the port between your thumb and the first two fingers of your nondominant hand.
- Using your dominant hand, aim the noncoring needle at the center of the device.
- Insert the needle perpendicular to the port septum.

*Picture this!*

### How to access a top-entry VAP

Insert the needle perpendicular to the port.

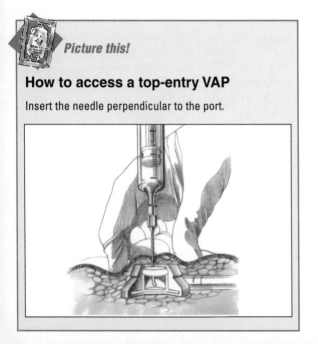

- Push the needle through the skin and septum until you reach the bottom of the reservoir.
- Check needle placement by aspirating for a blood return; if you can't obtain blood, remove the needle and repeat the procedure.
- Flush the device with normal saline solution.
- If you detect swelling or if the patient reports pain at the site, remove the needle and notify the doctor.

## What to consider

- Never use a traditional needle to access the system because it can core the septum, resulting in blood leakage and contact with air. A damaged port must be surgically removed immediately.
- An inability to obtain blood might indicate that the catheter is against the vessel wall. If you can't obtain a blood return after a second attempt, notify the doctor: A fibrin sleeve on the distal end of the catheter may be blocking the opening.

## Maintaining VAP infusions

## Administering a bolus injection by VAP

What to do

- Assemble the equipment.
- Attach a 10-ml syringe filled with saline solution to the end of the extension set.
- Remove all air.
- Attach the extension set to a Huber noncoring needle.
- Using sterile technique, clean the area over the port with alcohol followed by povidone-iodine solution.
- Insert the Huber noncoring needle into the skin over the port.
- Check for a blood return.
- Flush the port with saline solution, according to your facility's policy.
- Clamp the extension set.
- Remove the saline solution syringe.
- Connect the medication syringe to the extension set.
- Open the clamp and inject the prescribed drug.
- Examine the skin surrounding the needle for signs of infiltration, such as swelling or tenderness.

Make sure you have all your supplies when administering injections.

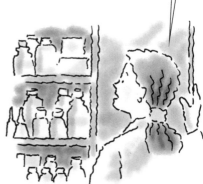

- When the injection is complete, clamp the extension set and remove the medication syringe.
- Open the clamp.
- Flush with 5 ml of saline solution after each drug injection to minimize drug incompatibility reactions.
- Flush with heparin solution, as your facility's policy directs.
- Document the injection according to your facility's policy; be sure to include:
  – the type of medication injected
  – the amount of injection
  – the time of the injection
  – the appearance of the site
  – the patient's tolerance of the procedure
  – any pertinent nursing interventions.

## What to consider

- Some facilities require flushing the port with heparin solution first; always check your facility's policy.
- Stop the injection if you note signs of infiltration and intervene appropriately.

# Administering a continuous VAP infusion

## What to do

- Assemble the equipment.
- Remove all the air from the extension set by priming it with an attached syringe of saline solution.
- Attach the extension set to a Huber noncoring needle.
- Flush the port system with saline solution.
- Clamp the extension set.
- Remove the syringe.
- Connect the administration set.
- Secure the connections with tape if necessary.
- Unclamp the extension set.
- Begin the infusion.
- Apply a transparent semipermeable dressing over the needle insertion site.
- Examine the site carefully for infiltration.
- When the solution container is empty, obtain a new I.V. solution container, as ordered, with primed I.V. tubing.
- Clamp the extension set.
- Remove the old I.V. tubing.
- Attach the new I.V. tubing with the solution container to the extension set.
- Open the clamps.
- Adjust the infusion rate.
- Document the infusion according to your facility's policy.

## What to consider

- If the patient complains of burning, stinging, or pain at the site, discontinue the infusion and intervene appropriately.

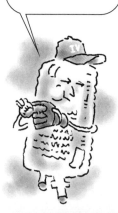

A continuous VAP infusion is kind of like a ball game with extra innings...You may need a reliever if the container has nothing left!

# Discontinuing a VAP infusion

*What to do*

- Stop the infusion.
- Clamp the extension set.
- Remove the I.V. tubing.
- Attach a 10-ml syringe filled with 5 ml of normal saline solution using sterile technique.
- Unclamp the extension set.
- Flush the device with the saline solution.
- Remove the saline solution syringe.
- Attach a 10-ml syringe filled with 5 ml of sterile heparin flush solution (100 units/ml).
- Flush the port with the heparin solution.
- Clamp the extension set.

# Removing a noncoring needle

## What to do

- Flush the port with heparin solution.
- Place the gloved index and middle fingers from your nondominant hand on either side of the port septum.
- Stabilize the port by pressing down with these two fingers, maintaining pressure until the needle is removed.
- Using your gloved, dominant hand, grasp the noncoring needle and pull it straight out of the port.
- Apply a dressing as indicated.

## What to consider

- If no more infusions are scheduled, remind the patient that he'll need a heparin flush in 4 weeks.

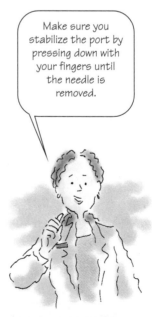

Make sure you stabilize the port by pressing down with your fingers until the needle is removed.

# Drawing blood from a VAP

## Syringe technique

### What to do

- Assemble the proper equipment.
- Attach the 10-ml syringe with 5 ml of saline solution to the noncoring needle and extension set.
- Remove all air.
- Palpate the area over the port to locate it.
- Access the port.
- Flush the VAP with 5 ml of saline solution.
- Withdraw at least 5 ml of blood.
- Clamp the extension set.
- Discard the syringe.
- Connect another 10-ml sterile syringe to the extension set.
- Unclamp the set.
- Aspirate the desired amount of blood into the 10-ml syringe.
- After obtaining the sample, clamp the extension set.
- Remove the syringe.
- Attach a 10-ml syringe filled with saline solution.
- Unclamp the extension set.
- Immediately flush the VAP with 20 ml of saline solution. (Solution concentrations and amounts may vary according to your facility's policy.)
- Clamp the extension set.
- Remove the saline syringe.
- Attach a sterile heparin-filled syringe.
- Perform the heparin flush procedure.
- Transfer the blood into appropriate blood sample tubes, label the tubes, and send them to the laboratory.

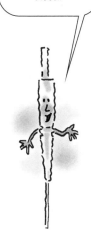

Don't forget, it's important to flush me out with heparin after drawing blood.

# Evacuated technique

## What to do

- Assemble the proper equipment.
- Apply the evacuated tube needle to the tube's holder.
- Attach the luer-lock injection cap to the noncoring needle extension set, using sterile technique.
- Remove all air from the set with the saline-filled syringe.
- Palpate the area over the port to locate it.
- Access the port.
- Flush the VAP with 5 ml of saline solution to ensure correct noncoring needle placement.
- Remove the saline solution syringe.
- Wipe the injection cap with an alcohol or a povidone-iodine swab.
- Insert the evacuated tube needle or needleless device into the injection cap.
- Insert the blood sample tube labeled "Discard" into the evacuated tube holder.
- Allow the tube to fill with blood.
- Remove the tube and discard.
- Insert another tube and allow it to fill with blood.

As with any project, make sure you have all the parts you'll need!

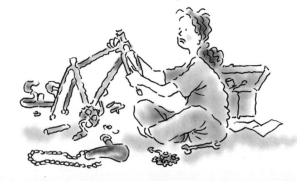

- Repeat this procedure until you obtain the desired amount of blood.
- Remove the evacuated tube needle or needleless device from the injection cap.
- Insert the 10-ml saline-filled syringe.
- Immediately flush the VAP with 10-ml of saline solution.
- Remove the syringe.
- Attach the heparin-filled syringe and needle.
- Perform the heparin flush procedure.
- Clamp the extension set.
- Transfer the blood into appropriate blood sample tubes, label the tubes and send them to the laboratory.

## What to consider

- If administering a bolus injection, use the syringe method to obtain the blood sample, but don't flush with heparin solution.

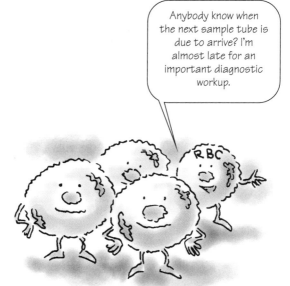

# Sampling during continuous infusion

## What to do

- Shut off the infusion.
- Clamp the extension set.
- Disconnect the extension set, maintaining sterile technique.
- Follow the procedure for obtaining a blood sample with a syringe, up to and including the saline solution flush procedure.
- After the catheter is flushed with saline solution, clamp the extension set.
- Remove the syringe.
- Reconnect the I.V. extension set.
- Unclamp the extension set.
- Adjust the flow rate.
- Transfer the blood into appropriate blood sample tubes, label the tubes, and send them to the laboratory.

## Managing complications of VAP therapy

## Extravasation

### What to look for
- Burning sensation or swelling in subcutaneous tissue

### What causes it
- Needle dislodged into subcutaneous tissue
- Needle incorrectly placed in VAP
- Needle position not confirmed
- Needle pulled out of septum
- Rupture of catheter along tunneled route

### What to do
- Stop the infusion.
- Don't remove the needle.
- Notify the doctor; prepare to administer an antidote if prescribed.

### How to prevent it
- Teach the patient how to access the device, verify its placement, and secure the needle before initiating the infusion.

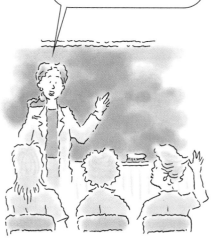

When teaching a patient to care for a VAP, explain, show, write it down, and ask her to demonstrate what she has learned.

*Smooth sailing*

## Troubleshooting common VAP problems

| What's wrong and why it happens | What to do |
| --- | --- |
| **Inability to flush or withdraw blood** | |
| • Kinked tubing or closed clamp | • Check the tubing or clamp. |
| • Incorrect needle placement<br>• Needle not advanced through septum | • Regain access to the device. |
| • Clot formation | • Assess patency by trying to flush the VAP.<br>• Notify the doctor; obtain an order for thrombolytic instillation.<br>• Teach the patient to recognize clot formation, to notify the doctor if it occurs, and to avoid forcibly flushing the VAP. |
| • Kinked catheter, catheter migration, port rotation | • Notify the doctor immediately.<br>• Tell the patient to notify the doctor or home care nurse if he has difficulty accessing the port. |

**Troubleshooting common VAP problems** (continued)

| What's wrong and why it happens | What to do |
|---|---|
| *Inability to palpate VAP* | |
| • Deeply implanted port | • Note the portal chamber scar. |
| | • Use the deep palpation technique. |
| | • Ask another nurse to try locating the VAP. |
| | • Use a 1½″ to 2″ noncoring needle to gain access to the VAP. |
| | • If you can't feel the port, don't attempt to access it. |

# Fibrin sheath formation

## What to look for
- Blocked port and catheter lumen
- Inability to flush port or administer infusion

## What causes it
- Adherence of platelets to the catheter

## What to do
- Notify the doctor and prepare to administer a thrombolytic agent.

## How to prevent it
- Use the port only to infuse fluids and medications; don't use the port to obtain blood samples.
- Administer only compatible substances through the port.

# Site infection and breakdown

## What to look for
- Erythema and warmth at the port site
- Fever
- Oozing or purulent drainage at the port site or VAP pocket

## What causes it
- Infected incision or VAP pocket
- Poor postoperative healing

## What to do
- Assess the port site daily for redness and drainage, and notify the doctor if present.
- Administer prescribed antibiotics.
- Apply warm soaks for 20 minutes four times per day.

## How to prevent it
- Teach the patient to inspect for and report any redness, swelling, drainage, or skin breakdown at the port site.

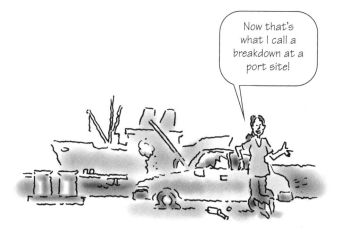

# Thrombosis

## What to look for
- Inability to flush the port or administer an infusion

## What causes it
- Frequent blood sampling
- Infusion of packed red blood cells (RBCs)

## What to do
- Notify the doctor, and obtain an order to administer a thrombolytic agent.

## How to prevent it
- Flush the VAP thoroughly immediately after obtaining a blood sample.
- Administer packed RBCs as a piggyback with saline solution, and use an infusion pump; flush with saline solution between units.

# I.V. medications

# 4

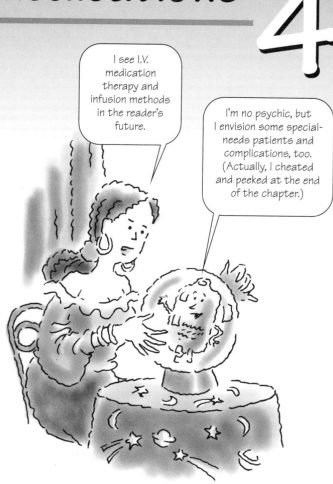

# Understanding I.V. medication therapy

## I.V. medication therapy basics

### Key facts

- I.V. medications may be given by direct injection, intermittent infusion, and continuous infusion.

### The pros

- Rapid response
- Effective absorption
- Accurate titration
- Less discomfort than I.M. injections
- Viable alternative to the oral route

### The cons

- Possible solution and drug incompatibilities
- Poor vascular access in some patients
- Potential for immediate adverse reactions

# Factors affecting drug compatibility

## Key facts

Drug compatibility may be affected by contact time, drug concentration, mixing order, pH, light, and temperature.

## What to consider

- Contact time
  – Incompatibility more likely the longer two or more drugs are together
- Drug concentration
  – Incompatibility more likely with higher drug concentrations
- Order of mixing
  – A concern when adding more than one drug to an I.V. solution because chemical changes occur after each drug is added
  – Drug normally compatible with a particular I.V. solution may be incompatible with a mixture of the same I.V. solution and other drugs
- pH
  – Incompatibility more likely if the drugs and solutions to be mixed have greatly differing pH values
- Light
  – Stability of certain drugs affected by prolonged exposure to light
- Temperature
  – Incompatibility more likely when the admixture reaches higher-than-normal temperatures (higher temperatures promote chemical reactions)

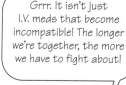

Grrr. It isn't just I.V. meds that become incompatible! The longer we're together, the more we have to fight about!

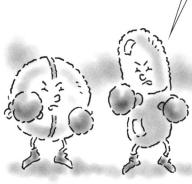

## What to do

- Verify drug compatibility times before administration.
- To prevent a high-concentration buildup, gently invert the container after adding each drug to evenly disperse it throughout the solution. Perform this step before starting an infusion and before adding another drug to the container.
- Verify the correct mixing order before starting (may prevent incompatibility).
- Before administration, verify that the solutions and drugs to be mixed have similar pH values. (The pH of each I.V. solution is listed on the manufacturer's label; the pH of each drug can be found on the package insert.)
- Store light-sensitive drugs in darkened storage areas or in protective plastic bags.
- Administer drugs that must be protected from light during administration, such as nitroprusside and amphotericin B, by wrapping the I.V. solution (but not the infusion tubing) in aluminum foil.
- Prepare the admixture immediately before administering it, if possible; if it must be prepared ahead of time, refrigerate it until needed.

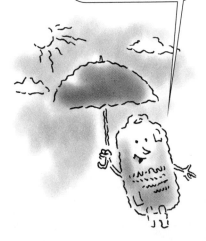

When it comes to light, I can sometimes be a sensitive guy who needs to be protected during storage and administration.

# Calculating I.V. drug dosages

## Key facts

- With some drugs (such as I.V. immune globulin), the dosage is based on the patient's weight in kilograms (2.2 lb = 1 kg).
  – Pounds to kilograms: divide the number of pounds by 2.2
- With other drugs (such as chemotherapeutic agents), the dosage is based on the patient's body surface area (BSA).
  – A nomogram may be used for determining BSA.

## Calculating administration rates

- Typically, an order for I.V. medication prescribes the number of milliliters to infuse over a specific period.
- To deliver the solution evenly, determine how many milliliters to give in 1 hour by dividing the total volume of the infusion by the number of hours the infusion is to take.

*Example:* The doctor orders the patient to receive 1,000 ml of dextrose 5% in half-normal saline solution every 8 hours. Before administering the solution, you divide 1,000 ml by 8 hours to determine that you must give 125 ml/hour.

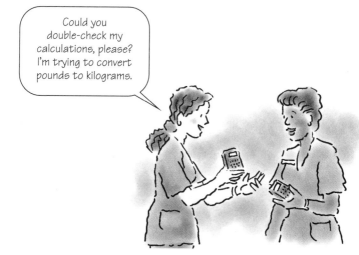

# Adding drugs

## What to do

### Adding a drug to an I.V. bottle

- Clean the rubber stopper or latex diaphragm with alcohol.
- Insert the needle (19G or 20G) of the medication-filled syringe into the center of the stopper or diaphragm, and inject the drug.
- Invert the bottle at least twice to ensure thorough mixing.
- Remove the latex diaphragm.
- Insert the administration spike.
- After injecting the drug, invert the bottle several times to ensure thorough mixing and to prevent a bolus effect.

### Adding a drug to an I.V. bag

- Insert the needle (19G or 20G and 1″ long) of the medication-filled syringe into the clean latex medication port.
- A short needle won't pierce the inner port seal, and a small-volume additive, such as insulin, will remain in the port.
- Inject the drug.
- After injecting the drug, gently invert the bag several times to ensure thorough mixing and to prevent a bolus effect.

### Adding a drug to an infusing solution

- If you have a choice, don't add a drug to an I.V. solution that's already infusing, as this may alter the drug concentration.
- Clamp the I.V. tubing.
- Take down the container.
- With the container upright, add the drug.
  – If you're adding the drug to a bottle, clean the rubber stopper with an alcohol swab, insert the needle through the stopper, and inject the drug.
  – If you're adding the drug to an I.V. bag, clean the rubber injection port with an alcohol swab before you inject the drug.
- After injecting the drug into the container, gently invert the container several times to ensure thorough mixing and to prevent a bolus effect.

## Comparing infusion methods

## Continuous infusion through a primary line

### Why it's done
- To maintain continuous serum levels if the infusion isn't likely to be stopped abruptly

### The pros
- Maintains steady serum levels
- Less risk of rapid shock and vein irritation because of the large volume of fluid diluting the drug

### The cons
- Risk of incompatibility increases with drug contact time
- Increased risk of undetected infiltration
- Restricts patient mobility

# Continuous infusion through a secondary line

## Why it's done

- To allow continuous infusion of two or more compatible admixtures administered at different rates
- To abruptly stop one admixture without infusing the remaining drug in the I.V. tubing

## The pros

- Allows the primary infusion and each secondary infusion to be given at different rates
- Allows the primary line to be totally shut off and kept on standby to maintain venous access in case the secondary line must be abruptly stopped
- Short contact time before infusion may allow the administration of incompatible admixtures — something not possible with long contact time

## The cons

- Can't be used for drugs with immediate incompatibility
- Increased risk of vein irritation or phlebitis from the increased number of drugs
- Use of multiple I.V. systems, especially with electronic pumps, can create physical barriers to patient care and limit patient mobility.

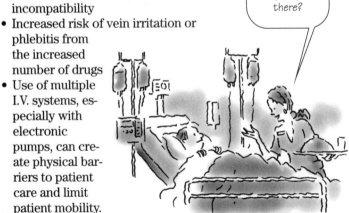

# Direct injection into a vein (no infusion line)

## Why it's done

- To administer a nonvesicant drug with a low risk of immediate adverse effects to a patient with no other I.V. needs (for example, outpatients requiring I.V. contrast injections for radiologic examinations or cancer patients receiving chemotherapeutic agents)

## The pros

- Eliminates the risk of complications from indwelling venipuncture devices
- Eliminates the inconvenience of an indwelling venipuncture device

## The cons

- Can be given only by a doctor or specially certified nurse
- Requires venipuncture, which can cause patient anxiety
- Requires two syringes — one to administer the medication and one to flush the vein after administration
- Risk of infiltration from steel needle
- Can't dilute drug or interrupt delivery if irritation occurs
- Risk of clotting with the administration of a drug over a long period and with a small volume

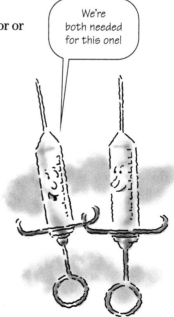

# Direct injection through an existing infusion line

## Why it's done

- To administer a drug that's incompatible with an I.V. solution and that must be given as a bolus injection
- To achieve immediate high blood levels (for example, regular insulin, dextrose 50%, atropine, antihistamines)
- To achieve an immediate drug effect in emergencies

## The pros

- Doesn't require time or authorization to perform venipuncture because the vein is already accessed
- Doesn't require needle puncture, which can cause patient anxiety
- Allows the use of I.V. solution to test the patency of the venipuncture device before drug administration
- Allows continued venous access in the case of adverse reactions
- Reduces the risk of infiltration with vesicant drugs because most continuous infusions are started with an over-the-needle catheter

## The cons

- Same inconveniences and complications risk (incompatibility, vein irritation, phlebitis) as those seen with indwelling venipuncture devices

# Intermittent infusion using the piggyback method

## Why it's done

- To administer drugs that are given over short periods at varying intervals (such as antibiotics and gastric-secretion inhibitors)

## The pros

- Avoids multiple needle injections required by the I.M. route
- Permits repeated administration of drugs through a single I.V. site
- Provides high drug blood levels for short periods without causing drug toxicity

## The cons

- At times, drug blood level may become too low to be clinically effective (such as when peak and trough times aren't considered in the drug order)

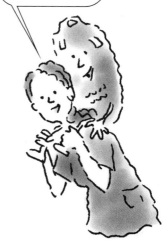

He ain't heavy...he's my piggyback method for intermittent I.V. infusion.

# Intermittent infusion using a saline lock

## Why it's done
- To provide constant venous access in a patient who doesn't need a continuous infusion

## The pros
- Provides venous access for patients with fluid restrictions
- Provides better patient mobility between doses
- Preserves veins by reducing the need for venipunctures
- Lowers cost if used with a limited number of drugs

## The cons
- Requires close monitoring during administration so the device can be flushed on completion

# Intermittent infusion using a volume-control set

## Why it's done
- To infuse a low volume of fluid
- To treat infants and children with cardiopulmonary problems (more prone to fluid overload)

## The pros
- Requires only one large-volume container
- Prevents fluid overload from a runaway infusion
- Allows the chamber to be reused

## The cons
- High cost
- High risk of contamination
- Requires manually closing the flow clamp if the set doesn't contain a membrane to block air passage when it's empty

For children with cardiopulmonary problems, turning down the volume on infusion reduces the risk of fluid overload.

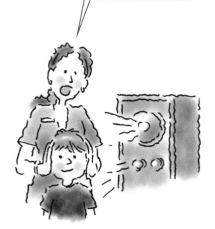

**Picture this!**

## Close look at a volume-control set

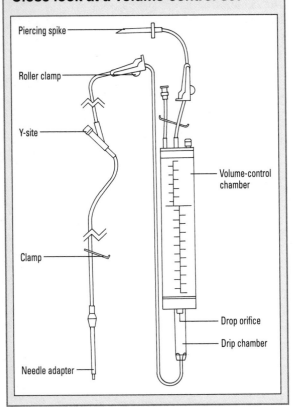

## Administering I.V. infusion therapy

## Injecting a drug directly into a vein

### What to do

- Assemble the appropriate equipment.
- Apply the tourniquet.
- Clean the I.V. site with a povidone-iodine or alcohol swab.
- Connect the syringe with medication to the small-vein needle.
- Push the plunger to expel the air.
- Select the largest suitable vein to allow for rapid dilution.
- Put on clean gloves.
- Insert the needle into the vein with the bevel up.
- Aspirate a small amount of blood to confirm needle placement.

### After the needle is properly placed

- Release the tourniquet.
- Place a short, narrow strip of tape or a transparent dressing over each needle wing to secure the device during administration.
- Inject the drug at an even rate as ordered.
- Gently aspirate the plunger at frequent intervals to reconfirm needle placement and ensure that all the medication is delivered.

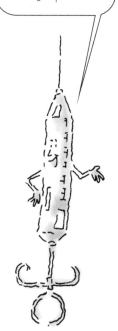

Before injecting that drug, better check that my needle is bevel up and in the right place.

## After the drug is injected

- Observe the patient for signs of adverse reactions (during and after the injection).
- Disconnect the medication syringe from the small-vein needle. Attach the syringe filled with saline solution to the needle, and flush the device to ensure the complete delivery of all medication.
- Remove the venipuncture device, and immediately place a sterile pressure dressing over the I.V. site.
- Dispose of contaminated hazardous equipment where appropriate.
- If your patient needs further I.V. therapy — or if the drug can cause an immediate adverse reaction — consider obtaining an order for an indwelling access device.

# Injecting a drug directly into an existing line

## What to do

- Assemble the appropriate equipment.
- Check the I.V. site for redness, tenderness, edema, or leakage.
- If you detect signs of complications, change the site before you administer the drug.
- If the new drug and the existing infusate are compatible, keep the infusion running.
- If the new drug isn't compatible with the infusate but is compatible with saline solution, use a saline-filled syringe to flush the line before injecting the drug.
- Invert the syringe, and gently push the plunger to remove all air.
- Using an alcohol swab, clean the rubber cap of the injection port closest to the venous access device.

### After initial preparations

- Stabilize the injection port with one hand and insert the needleless device (or needle) through the center of the rubber cap.
- Don't force the insertion; if you feel resistance, insert the device at a different angle.
- Inject the drug at an even rate as ordered; never inject so fast that you stop the primary infusion or allow the drug to flow back into the tubing.
- Observe the patient for signs of a reaction during and after the injection.
- Withdraw the needleless device (or needle) and reestablish the desired flow rate.

# Using a saline lock

## What to do

- Assemble the appropriate equipment.
- Attach the minibag to the administration set.
- Prime the tubing with the drug solution.
- Secure the needleless device to the I.V. tubing device.
- Prime the needleless device with the drug solution.
- Using an alcohol swab, clean the cap on the saline lock.
- Stabilize the saline lock with the thumb and index finger of your nondominant hand.

### After the saline lock is stabilized

- Insert the needleless device of one of the syringes containing flush solution into the center of the injection cap.
- Don't force the insertion; if you feel resistance, insert the device at a different angle.
- Pull back on the plunger slightly and watch for blood return. If blood appears, begin to slowly inject the flush solution.
- If you feel resistance or if the patient complains of pain or discomfort, stop immediately; the venous access device should be replaced.
- If you don't feel resistance, watch for signs of infiltration as you slowly inject the flush solution.
- If you note signs of infiltration, remove the venous access device and insert a new device in a new location; if you don't note signs of infiltration, you're ready to give the medication.
- Insert the needleless device attached to the administration set into the saline lock.
- Regulate the drip rate and infuse the medication as ordered.

### Discontinuing the infusion

- Close the I.V. flow clamp.
- Withdraw the needleless device.
- Clean the injection cap and flush the saline lock again.

# Tips for adding medications

### What to do

- When adding medications to a volume-control set, check for an immediately visible incompatibility—especially if you're using multiple lines.
- To prevent confusion when using multiple secondary lines, don't let them become tangled.
- Tag the lines below the drip chamber and at the connection site to the primary line; this clearly identifies the source and tubing connection for each drug.
- When possible, use a pump to achieve more accurate dosage control.
- Put a time strip on the secondary container to help monitor the administration rate.
- Maintain a secure, patent venous access device.
- To avoid interrupting drug therapy when you change the I.V. site, establish the new site before disconnecting the old one.
- Firmly stabilize the connection to the primary tubing with tape or a locking device to prevent dislodgment.

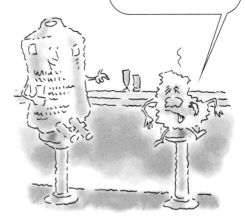

# Infusing medication through a secondary line

## What to do

- Attach the administration set to the solution container and prime the tubing with the I.V. solution.
- Attach the administration set to the pump, if appropriate.
- Secure the needleless device (if one isn't available, use a 20G 1″ needle) to the administration set.
- Prime the device with the I.V. solution.
- Place labels with the name of the drug under the drip chamber and at the end of the tubing.
- Clean the injection port on the primary tubing with an alcohol swab.

### When the injection port is clean

- Insert the full length of the needleless adapter into the center of the injection port.
- Regulate the drop rate of the secondary solution and adjust the rate of the primary solution.
- Frequently monitor the patient and the infusion rate.
- When the secondary infusion is completed, remove the needleless device from the injection port.
- Adjust the flow rate of the primary solution.

# Patient-controlled analgesia

## Key facts

- Allows the patient to self-administer medication by pressing a button on a handheld controller that's connected to a pump
- Must be programmed to deliver specified doses at predetermined time intervals before use
- Uses a lockout time to prevent the patient from accidentally overdosing
  – Lockout time between doses is usually 6 to 10 minutes, but can be longer
  – Lockout interval for I.V. boluses is set as prescribed

## Why it's used

- To provide parenteral analgesia
- To enhance postoperative pain management
- To enhance pain management in chronic diseases

## The pros

- Eliminates the need for I.M. analgesics
- Provides individualized pain relief
- Gives the patient a sense of control over his pain
- Allows the patient to sleep at night while minimizing daytime drowsiness

## The cons

- May cause respiratory depression; routine monitoring of the patient's respiratory rate is required
- May lower blood pressure
- Requires the patient to be mentally alert and able to understand and comply with instructions
- Restrictions include patients with a limited respiratory reserve and those with a history of drug abuse, chronic sedative or tranquilizer use, an analgesic allergy, or a psychiatric disorder

## Administering I.V. drugs to pediatric patients

## Pediatric infusion basics

### Key facts

- Neonates, infants, and small children have precise fluid requirements that should be kept in mind when giving I.V. medications.
  - Small children can't tolerate the large amount of fluid recommended for diluting many drugs.
  - Because the drug dosage is based on the child's weight, each patient has a different normal dosing.
- The most common method of giving I.V. drugs to pediatric patients is by intermittent infusion using a volume-control set.
- For drug dosages based on BSA, a nomogram may be used.

### What to do

- Explain the procedure to the child and parent; prepare the child for drug administration that may cause discomfort.
- Make sure that no drug remains in the I.V. tubing before you change it.
- Keep flow-control clamps out of the child's reach.
- Use tamper-proof pumps so the child can't change the rate inadvertently.
- Be especially careful to protect the I.V. site from accidental dislodgment or contamination; in many cases, a child's venipuncture device must stay in place longer than an adult's.

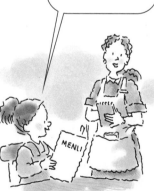

I'd like the small apple juice...you know I can't tolerate large amounts.

# Syringe pump

### Key facts

- Especially useful for giving intermittent I.V. medications to pediatric patients
- Provides the greatest control for small-volume infusions
- Must be tamper-proof, have a built-in guard against uncontrolled flow rates, and have an alarm sensitive to low-pressure occlusion
- Should operate accurately with syringe sizes from 5 to 60 ml using low-volume tubing

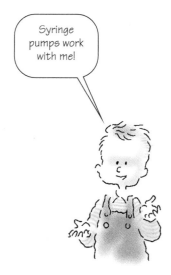

Syringe pumps work with me!

## Administering I.V. drugs to elderly patients

## Elderly I.V. basics

### Key facts

- Elderly patients with chronic conditions commonly need multiple medications, which requires careful monitoring for drug interactions.
- Close monitoring is required for patients receiving medications that cause renal toxicity.
- Accurate recording of the patient's intake and output—including all fluids given for I.V. drug administration—is a priority.
- Careful, individualized dosage adjustments are a priority because aging can enhance or reduce medication effects.

### What to do

- When administering an I.V. analgesic to an elderly patient, watch closely for signs of respiratory depression or central nervous system depression, including confusion.
- Carefully assess the I.V. site for signs and symptoms of infiltration and phlebitis, which are more prominent in elderly patients because of their fragile veins.
- When diluting a drug in a larger volume than normal (may be necessary because many I.V. drugs are irritating to fragile veins), monitor the patient carefully for signs of fluid overload (elderly patients are prone to this).
- If necessary, restart the infusion before you give a medication I.V.
- When inserting a venous access device, use tape minimally to prevent trauma to the elderly patient's fragile skin.

## Managing complications of I.V. medication therapy

### Circulatory overload

#### Key facts
- Can occur when too much I.V. solution is infused too quickly
- Can also be a frequent complication of I.V. therapy in patients with heart failure or renal disease and in elderly patients
- Prevention includes the careful monitoring of the rate and volume of all I.V. infusions

#### What to look for
- Crackles
- Increased blood pressure
- Jugular vein distention or engorgement
- Positive fluid balance
- Respiratory distress

#### What to do
- Stop the infusion.
- Place the patient in semi-Fowler's position as tolerated.
- Reduce the patient's anxiety.
- Administer oxygen as ordered.
- Notify the doctor.
- Administer diuretics as ordered.

#### How to prevent it
- Use a pump controller for elderly or immunocompromised patients.
- Recheck the fluid requirements calculations.
- Monitor the rate and volume of the infusion frequently.

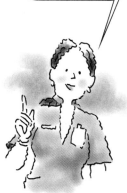

Stop the insanity—or at least the infusion! When you observe signs of fluid overload, stopping the infusion of the fluid is priority-one!

# Extravasation

## Key facts
- Involves infiltration of irritating fluids, resulting in damage to surrounding tissues
- Can occur when a vein is punctured or when there's leakage around an I.V. site
- May result in severe local tissue damage if vesicant (blistering) drugs or fluids extravasate

## What to look for
- Blanching
- Burning or discomfort at the I.V. site (but may be painless)
- Cool skin around the I.V. site
- Slow or continuing flow rate, even when the vein is occluded
- Swelling at and above the I.V. site
- Tight feeling at the I.V. site

## What to do
- Remove the venipuncture device.
- Notify the doctor.
- Monitor the patient's pulse and capillary refill time.

## How to prevent it
- Administer drugs by slow I.V. push through a free-flowing I.V. line or by small-volume infusion (50 to 100 ml).
- Monitor the infusion site for erythema or infiltration; tell the patient to report burning, stinging, pain, or a sensation of sudden "heat" at the site.
- Use a transparent, semipermeable dressing to allow frequent inspection of the I.V. site.
- After drug administration, instill several milliliters of $D_5W$ or normal saline solution to flush the drug from the vein and preclude drug leakage when the catheter is removed.

## When giving vesicants

- Strictly adhere to proper administration techniques.
- Don't use an existing I.V. line unless its patency is assured.
- Use a distal vein that allows successive venipunctures.
- Avoid using the back of the hand, where tendon and nerve damage from possible extravasation is more likely.
- Avoid the wrist and fingers (they're hard to immobilize) and areas having previous damage or poor circulation.
- Always start the infusion with $D_5W$ or normal saline solution.

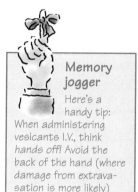

**Memory jogger**

Here's a handy tip: When administering vesicants I.V., think *hands off!* Avoid the back of the hand (where damage from extravasation is more likely) and the wrist and fingers (which are hard to immobilize).

- Check for infiltration before giving the medication.
- Give vesicants last when multiple drugs are ordered.
- If possible, avoid using an infusion pump to administer vesicants; a pump will continue the infusion if infiltration occurs.

# Hypersensitivity

## Key facts
- Occurs when a medication is administered to a patient who has a history of hypersensitivity to that medication, or develops hypersensitivity at the first administration

## What to look for
- Anaphylactic reaction
- Bronchospasm
- Itching, urticarial rash
- Tearing eyes, runny nose
- Wheezing

## What to do
- Stop the infusion immediately.
- Maintain a patent airway.
- Administer antihistaminic steroid, anti-inflammatory, and antipyretic medications as ordered.
- Give 0.2 to 0.5 ml of 1:1000 aqueous epinephrine subcutaneously; repeat at 3-minute intervals and as needed.
- Monitor the patient's vital signs.

## How to prevent it
- Obtain the patient's allergy history and be aware of cross allergies.
- Assist with test dosing, and document new allergies.
- Monitor the patient carefully during the first 15 minutes of the administration of a new drug.
- Before you administer an I.V. medication, take steps to find out if your patient may be prone to hypersensitivity.

# Infiltration

## Key facts

- Commonly results from improper placement or dislodgment of the catheter, allowing I.V. fluids and medications to permeate the surrounding tissue
- May occur in elderly patients because of their thin, fragile veins
- Risk increases when venous access device remains in the vein for more than 2 days or when the tip is positioned near a flexion area

## What to look for

- Blanching
- Burning
- Cool skin around the I.V. site
- Slow or continuing flow rate, even when the vein is occluded
- Swelling at and above the I.V. site
- Tight feeling at the I.V. site

## What to do

- Stop the infusion and remove the device.
- Check the patient's pulse and capillary refill time.
- Restart the I.V. catheter in a different location and restart the infusion.
- Document the patient's condition and your interventions.

## How to prevent it

- Check the I.V. site frequently.
- Don't obscure the area above the I.V. site with tape.

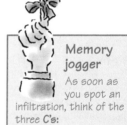

**Memory jogger**

As soon as you spot an infiltration, think of the three C's:

Cut off (the infusion)

Counteract (effects of the drug)

Contain (the affected area).

# Phlebitis

## Key facts

- Characterized by painful inflammation along the venous path in which the cannula is placed
- A common complication of I.V. therapy, usually associated with drugs or solutions that are acidic or alkaline or that have high osmolarity
- Contributing factors include vein trauma during insertion, using a vein that's too small, using a vascular access device that's too large, and prolonged use of the same I.V. site
- Can follow any infusion—or even an injection of a single drug—but more common after continuous infusions
- Typically develops 2 to 3 days after the vein is exposed to the drug or solution
- Develops more rapidly in distal veins than in the larger veins close to the heart
- Generally not caused by drugs given by direct injection and administered at the correct dilution and rate

---

### Classifying phlebitis

According to the 2000 Intravenous Nurses Society Standards of Practice, the degrees of phlebitis are classified as:

0 = no clinical symptoms

1 = erythema with or without pain

2 = pain with erythema or edema

3 = pain with erythema or edema, streak formation, and palpable venous cord

4 = pain with erythema or edema, streak formation, palpable venous cord greater than 1" (2.5 cm) in length, and purulent drainage.

- Can occur after one or more injections of phenytoin or diazepam given at the same I.V. site (these drugs are frequently given by direct injection)
- Commonly develops when irritating I.V. drugs (erythromycin, tetracycline, nafcillin, vancomycin, amphotericin B) are piggybacked
- May be caused by large doses of potassium chloride (40 mEq/L or more), amino acids, dextrose solutions (10% or more), or multivitamins

## What to look for

- Elevated temperature
- Hard vein on palpation
- Puffy area over the vein
- Redness or tenderness at the tip of the device
- Left untreated, may produce exudate at the I.V. site, accompanied by elevated white blood cell count and fever
- Can also produce pain at the I.V. site, but a lack of pain doesn't eliminate the possibility of phlebitis

## What to do

- Stop the infusion.
- Remove the venipuncture device.
- Apply warm soaks.
- Elevate the extremity if edema is present.
- Document the patient's condition and your interventions.
- Insert a new I.V. catheter using a larger vein or a smaller device.
- Restart the infusion in another limb.

## How to prevent it

- Use a large vein for irritating solutions.
- Tape the device securely to prevent movement.
- Use a small-gauge device for smaller veins to ensure adequate blood flow.

# Speed shock

## Key facts

- A systemic reaction that may occur when I.V. infusions are administered too quickly

## What to look for

- Cardiac arrest
- Flushed face
- Headache
- Irregular pulse
- Shock
- Syncope
- Tightness in chest

## What to do

- Stop the infusion.
- Call the doctor.
- Administer $D_5W$ at a keep-vein-open rate.

## How to prevent it

- Check the infusion guidelines before administering a drug; administer I.V. fluids at the prescribed rate.
- Never speed up a medication infusion.
- Use a pump for precise I.V. delivery.
- Dilute the drug with a compatible solution.

Save the speed for the racetrack! I.V. infusions that are given too quickly can cause speed shock.

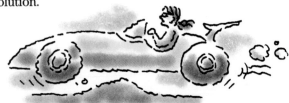

# Systemic infection

## Key facts
- Considered a serious complication of I.V. therapy
- More common in centrally placed vascular access devices than in those placed peripherally

## What to look for
- Fever, chills for no apparent reason
- Malaise for no apparent reason

## What to do
- Stop the infusion.
- Notify the doctor.
- Remove the device.
- Culture the site and device.
- Administer medications as prescribed.
- Monitor the patient's vital signs.

## How to prevent it
- Use meticulous aseptic technique when handling solutions and tubing, inserting the venipuncture device, and discontinuing the infusion.
- Secure all connections.
- Change the I.V. solution, tubing, and venipuncture device at the recommended times.
- Use transparent dressings over the vascular access insertion site to keep the site clean and allow moisture to escape, which discourages bacterial growth.

# Venous spasm

## Key facts
- Characterized by sudden contraction of the vein
- Can result from infusing cold I.V. solutions or irritating medications, or from a traumatic venipuncture

## What to look for
- Blanched skin over the vein
- Pain along the vein
- Sluggish flow rate when the clamp is completely open

## What to do
- Apply warm soaks over the vein and surrounding tissue.
- Slow the flow rate.

## How to prevent it
- Use a blood warmer for blood or packed red blood cells.
- Allow I.V. solutions and medications to come to room temperature before administration.
- Dilute irritating medications (calcium chloride, vancomycin) before administration.

> Your patient will pay the price if you don't follow these steps for preventing venous spasm.

# Transfusions 5

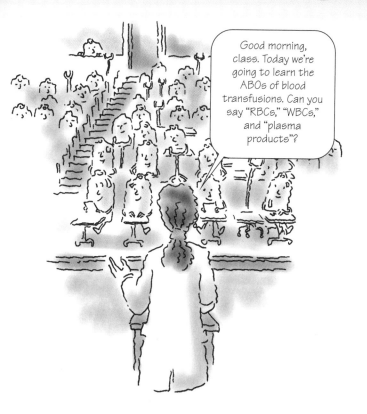

## Comparing cellular products

# Whole blood

### Key facts
- Complete (pure) blood
- Volume: 500 ml

### Why it's used
- To restore blood volume in hemorrhaging, trauma, or burn patients

### What to do
- Use a straight-line or Y-type I.V. set.
- Reduce the risk of transfusion reaction by adding a microfilter to remove platelets.
- Warm blood if giving a large quantity.
- Avoid giving whole blood when the patient can't tolerate the circulating volume.

### What to consider
- Crossmatching is ABO-identical:
  - Group A receives A
  - Group B receives B
  - Group AB receives AB
  - Group O receives O
  - Rh type must match
- Whole blood is commonly used in emergency treatment, but is seldom administered in nonemergency situa-

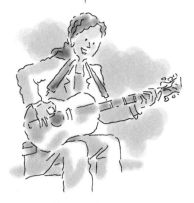

"...Wanna whole lotta blood...wanna whole lotta blood...."

## Blood type compatibility

Precise typing and crossmatching of donor and recipient blood helps avoid transfusing incompatible blood, which can be fatal. This chart shows ABO compatibility for recipient and donor.

| Blood group | Antibodies present in plasma | Compatible red blood cells | Compatible plasma |
|---|---|---|---|
| *Recipient* | | | |
| 0 | Anti-A and anti-B | 0 | 0, A, B, AB |
| A | Anti-B | A, 0 | A, AB |
| B | Anti-A | B, 0 | B, AB |
| AB | Neither anti-A nor anti-B | AB, A, B, 0 | AB |
| *Donor* | | | |
| 0 | Anti-A and anti-B | 0, A, B, AB | 0 |
| A | Anti-B | A, AB | A, 0 |
| B | Anti-A | B, AB | B, 0 |
| AB | Neither anti-A nor anti-B | AB | AB, A, B, 0 |

tions because its components can be extracted and administered separately.

- Whole blood may be infused rapidly in emergencies, but the rate should be adjusted to the patient's condition and the transfusion order; the blood shouldn't be infused for longer than 4 hours.

# Packed RBCs

## Key facts

- Same red blood cell (RBC) mass as whole blood, with 80% of the plasma removed
- Volume: 250 ml

## Why it's used

- To restore or maintain oxygen-carrying capacity
- To correct anemia and surgical blood loss
- To increase RBC mass

## What to do

- Use a straight-line or Y-type I.V. set.
- Infuse rapidly in emergencies or as ordered, but adjust the rate to the patient's condition and the transfusion order.
- Don't infuse for more than 4 hours.

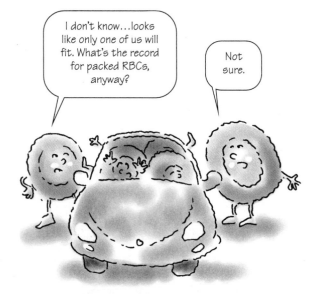

## What to consider

- Crossmatching:
  - Group A receives A or O
  - Group B receives B or O
  - Group AB receives AB, A, B, or O
  - Group O receives O
  - Rh type must match
- RBCs have the same oxygen-carrying capacity as whole blood, minimizing the hazard of volume overload.
- Using packed RBCs avoids the potassium and ammonia buildup that sometimes occurs in the plasma of stored blood.
- Packed RBCs shouldn't be used for anemic conditions correctable by nutrition or drug therapy.

# Leukocyte-poor RBCs

## Key facts
- Same as packed RBCs except leukocytes (70%) are removed
- Volume: 200 ml

## Why it's used
- To restore or maintain oxygen-carrying capacity
- To correct anemia and surgical blood loss
- To increase RBC mass
- To prevent febrile reactions from leukocyte antibodies
- To treat patients who are immunosuppressed

## What to do
- Use a straight-line or Y-type I.V. set; may require a microaggregate filter (40-micron) for hard-spun, leukocyte-poor RBCs.
- Infuse over 1½ to 4 hours.

## What to consider
- Crossmatching:
  - Group A receives A or O
  - Group B receives B or O
  - Group AB receives AB, A, B, or O
  - Group O receives O
  - Rh type must match
- Cells expire 24 hours after washing.
- RBCs have the same oxygen-carrying capacity as whole blood, minimizing the hazard of volume overload.
- Leukocyte-poor RBCs shouldn't be used to treat anemic conditions correctable by nutrition or drug therapy.

# WBCs (leukocytes)

## Key facts
- Whole blood with all RBCs and 80% of plasma removed
- Volume: usually 150 ml

## Why it's used
- To treat a patient with life-threatening granulocytopenia who isn't responding to antibiotics

## What to do
- Use a straight-line I.V. set with a standard in-line blood filter.
- Give 1 unit daily for 5 days or until the infection clears.
- To prevent possible fever and chills from white blood cell (WBC) infusion, premedicate the patient with antihistamines, acetaminophen, steroids, or meperidine.
- Because reactions are common, administer slowly over 2 to 4 hours.
- Check the patient's vital signs every 15 minutes throughout the transfusion.
- Give the transfusion in conjunction with antibiotics to treat infection.
- Agitate the container to prevent delivery of a bolus dose of WBCs.

## What to consider
- Crossmatching:
  - Group A receives A or O
  - Group B receives B or O
  - Group AB receives AB, A, B, or O
  - Group O receives O
  - Rh type must match
- WBCs are preferably human leukocyte antigen (HLA)—compatible, but compatibility isn't necessary unless the patient is HLA-sensitized from previous transfusions.

# Platelets

## Key facts
- Platelet sediment from RBCs or plasma
- Volume: 35 to 50 ml/unit; 1 unit of platelets = $7 \times 10^7$ platelets

## Why it's used
- To treat thrombocytopenia caused by decreased platelet production, increased platelet destruction, or massive transfusion of stored blood
- To treat acute leukemia and marrow aplasia
- To restore platelet count in a preoperative patient with a count of 100,000/µl or less

## What to do
- Use a blood component drip administration set.
- Infuse 100 ml over 15 minutes.
- Administer at 150 ml/hour to 200 ml/hour, or as rapidly as the patient can tolerate; don't exceed 4 hours.
- Don't use a microaggregate filter.
- Premedicate with antipyretics and antihistamines in patients with a history of platelet reaction.
- Avoid administering platelets when the patient has a fever.

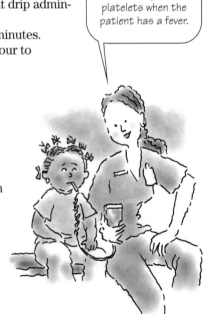

Don't give platelets when the patient has a fever.

## What to consider

- Crossmatching: ABO compatibility isn't necessary but is preferable with repeated platelet transfusions; Rh type match is preferred.
- Platelet transfusions aren't usually indicated for conditions of accelerated platelet destruction, such as idiopathic thrombocytopenic purpura or drug-induced thrombocytopenia.
- A blood platelet count may be ordered 1 hour after platelet transfusion to determine platelet transfusion increments.

# Administering transfusions

## Preparing for transfusion

### What to do

- Obtain whole blood or packed RBCs within 30 minutes of transfusion time.
- Check, recheck, and verify the type, Rh, and expiration date of the blood or cellular component.
- Double-check that you're giving the right blood or cellular component to the right patient by comparing the name and number on the patient's wristband with those on the blood bag.
- Check the blood bag identification number and ABO blood group and Rh compatibility.
- Inspect the blood or cellular component for abnormal color, clumping of RBCs, gas bubbles, and extraneous material that might indicate bacterial contamination; return the bag to the blood bank if you see any of these signs.
- Prepare the equipment.
- Use a Y-type blood administration set; blood and saline are both connected and can be clamped without opening the system.
- Close all the clamps on the set.
- Insert the spike of the line you're using for the normal saline solution into the bag of normal saline solution.
- Open the port on the blood bag.
- Insert the spike of the line you're using to administer the blood or cellular component into the port.

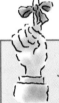

**Memory jogger**

Before beginning a transfusion, remember to check the four rights of blood transfusion:

- the right **blood or cellular component**
- the right **ABO group**
- the right **Rh compatibility**
- the right **patient.**

- Hang the bag of normal saline solution and blood or cellular component on the I.V. pole.
- Open the clamp on the line of normal saline solution.
- Squeeze the drip chamber until it's half full of normal saline solution.
- Remove the adapter cover at the tip of the blood administration set.
- Open the main flow clamp.
- Prime the tubing with normal saline solution.
- Close the clamp, and recap the adapter.

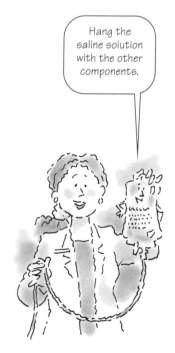

Hang the saline solution with the other components.

# Transfusing blood or cellular component

## What to do

- Take the patient's vital signs to serve as baseline values.
- Recheck the patient's vital signs after 15 minutes (or according to your facility's policy).
- If the patient doesn't have an I.V. device in place, perform a venipuncture, using a 20G or larger catheter.
- Attach the prepared blood administration set to the venous access device using a needleless connection, and flush it with normal saline solution.
- When using a Y-type set, open the clamp on the normal saline solution line and the main flow clamp.
- When preparing to infuse whole blood or WBCs, gently invert the bag several times before administering to mix the cells. (During the transfusion, gently agitate the bag to prevent the viscous cells from settling.)
- Begin transfusion after you've flushed the venous access device.
- Adjust the flow clamp closest to the patient to deliver a slow rate (usually about 20 gtt/minute) for the first 10 to 30 minutes.
- Allow the transfusion to run until completed, but no longer than 4 hours.
- Discard unused blood, or return it to the blood bank, following your facility's protocol.

## What to consider

- The type of blood product and the patient's clinical condition determine the rate of transfusion.
  - A unit of RBCs may be given over a period of 1 to 4 hours.
  - Platelets and coagulation factors may be given more quickly than RBCs and granulocytes.
- Blood shouldn't be transfused for longer than 4 hours because the risk of contamination and sepsis increases. Be sure to discard or return to the blood bank blood or blood products not given within 4 hours (or according to facility policy).

# Transfusing plasma or plasma fractions

## What to do

- Obtain the patient's baseline vital signs.
- Flush the patient's venous access device with normal saline solution.
- Attach the plasma, fresh frozen plasma (FFP), albumin, factor VIII concentrate, prothrombin complex, platelets, or cryoprecipitate to the patient's venous access device.
- Begin the transfusion.
- Adjust the flow rate as ordered.
- Take the patient's vital signs.
- Assess the patient frequently for signs or symptoms of a transfusion reaction, such as fever, chills, or nausea.
- After the infusion, flush the line with 20 to 30 ml of normal saline solution.
- Disconnect the I.V. line.
- If therapy is to continue, resume the prescribed infusate and adjust the flow rate as ordered.
- Record the type and amount of plasma or plasma fraction administered, duration of transfusion, the patient's baseline vital signs, and adverse reactions.

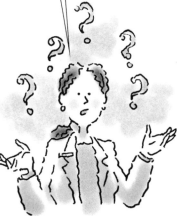

Transfusing fractions...I must be on the math unit, not the intensive care unit.

# Monitoring a blood transfusion

## Key facts

- Careful monitoring is needed to prevent transfusion reactions.

## What to do

- Record the patient's vital signs before the transfusion, 15 minutes after the start of the transfusion, and just after the transfusion is complete.
- Record the patient's vital signs more frequently if warranted by his condition and transfusion history, or your facility's policy.
- Always use sterile normal saline solution, set up as a primary line along with the transfusion.
- Observe for signs and symptoms of a hemolytic reaction.
- Act promptly to open the airway if your patient develops signs of an allergic reaction or anaphylaxis.

## What to consider

- Most hemolytic reactions occur within the first 30 minutes of a transfusion; monitor your patient carefully during this time.
- Dyspnea, flushing, and chest pain (with or without vomiting and diarrhea) after transfusion of the first few milliliters of blood may be signs of an anaphylactic reaction.

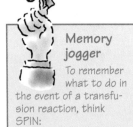

**Memory jogger**

To remember what to do in the event of a transfusion reaction, think SPIN:

**S**top the infusion.

**P**ulse and other vital signs need checking.

**I**nfuse normal saline solution.

**N**otify the doctor.

# Using a pressure cuff

## Why it's used
- To achieve rapid blood replacement

## What to do
- Insert your hand into the top of the pressure cuff sleeve.
- Pull the blood bag up through the center opening.
- Hang the blood bag loop on the hook provided with the sleeve.
- Hang the pressure cuff and blood bag on the I.V. pole.
- Open the flow clamp on the tubing.
- To set the flow rate, turn the screw clamp on the pressure cuff counterclockwise.
- Compress the pressure bulb of the cuff to inflate the bag until you achieve the desired flow rate.
- Turn the screw clamp clockwise to maintain this constant flow rate.
- Check the flow rate regularly, and adjust the pressure in the pressure cuff as necessary to maintain a consistent rate; as the blood bag empties, the pressure decreases.

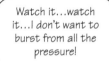

Watch it...watch it...I don't want to burst from all the pressure!

## What to consider
- Don't allow the cuff needle to exceed 300 mm Hg; excessively high pressure can cause hemolysis and damage the component container or rupture the blood bag.
- Watch the patient closely; increasing the pressure also increases the speed at which complications, such as infiltration, can occur.

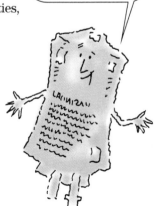

# Transfusion precautions

## What to do

- Don't add medications to the blood bag.
- Never give blood products without checking the order against the blood bag label—the only way to tell if the request form has been stamped with the wrong name. (Most life-threatening reactions occur when this step is omitted.)
- Don't transfuse the blood product if you discover a discrepancy in the blood number, blood slip type, or patient identification number.
- Don't piggyback blood into the port of an existing infusion set. Most solutions, including dextrose in water, are incompatible with blood; administer blood only with normal saline solution.
- Don't hesitate to stop the transfusion if your patient:
  – shows changes in his vital signs
  – is dyspneic or restless
  – develops chills, hematuria, or pain in his flank, chest, or back.
- Keep the vein open with a slow infusion of normal saline solution; call the doctor and the laboratory.
- If the blood bag empties before the next one arrives, administer normal saline solution slowly.

## Comparing plasma products

## Fresh frozen plasma

### Key facts
- Uncoagulated plasma separated from RBCs; rich in coagulation factors V, VIII, and IX
- Volume: 200 to 250 ml

### Why it's used
- To expand plasma volume
- To treat postsurgical hemorrhage or shock
- To correct an undetermined coagulation factor deficiency
- To replace a specific factor when that factor alone isn't available
- To correct factor deficiencies resulting from hepatic disease

### What to do
- Use a straight-line I.V. set and administer FFP as rapidly as tolerated.

### What to consider
- ABO compatibility isn't necessary but is preferable with repeated plasma transfusions; Rh type match is preferred.
- Large-volume transfusions of FFP may require correction for hypocalcemia. Citric acid in FFP binds calcium.

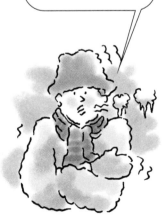

Brrr! FFP is actually uncoagulated plasma that's been separated from RBCs.

# Albumin 5% (buffered saline) and albumin 25% (salt-poor)

## Key facts

- Human albumin (a small plasma protein separated from plasma)
- Commonly given as a volume expander until crossmatching for whole blood is complete
- Volume 5% = 12.5 g/250 ml
- Volume 25% = 12.5 g/50 ml

## Why it's used

- To replace volume in the treatment of shock from burns, trauma, surgery, or infection
- To prevent marked hemoconcentration
- To treat hypoproteinemia (with or without edema)

> Overload of any kind is never good news for me!

## What to do

- Use a straight-line I.V. set.
- Administer at a rate and volume according to the patient's condition and response.
- Administer cautiously in patients with cardiac or pulmonary disease because of the risk of heart failure from circulatory overload.

## What to consider

- Don't mix albumin with protein hydrolysates or alcohol solutions. These solutions are incompatible with blood.
- Cross-typing isn't necessary.
- Reactions to albumin (fever, chills, nausea) are rare.
- Albumin is contraindicated as an expander in patients with severe anemia.

# Factor VIII

## Key facts

- Cold, insoluble portion of plasma recovered from FFP
- Volume: approximately 30 ml (freeze-dried)

## Why it's used

- To treat a patient with hemophilia A
- To control bleeding associated with factor VIII deficiency
- To replace fibrinogen or factor VIII

## What to do

- Use the manufacturer-supplied administration set; administer with a filter.
- Administer I.V. as rapidly as tolerated, but don't exceed 6 ml/minute; monitor the patient's pulse rate while infusing.

## What to consider

- ABO compatibility is preferable but not necessary.
- The standard dose recommended for treatment of acute bleeding episodes in hemophilia is 15 to 20 units/kg; the half-life of factor VIII (8 to 10 hours) necessitates repeat transfusions at these intervals to maintain normal levels.

# Factors II, VII, IX, and X complex

## Key facts

- Lyophilized, commercially prepared solution drawn from pooled plasma

## Why it's used

- To treat a congenital factor V deficiency and other bleeding disorders resulting from an acquired deficiency of factors II, VII, IX, and X

## What to do

- Use a straight-line I.V. set.
- Administer the dosage based on the desired level and the patient's body weight.
- Perform coagulation assays, as ordered, before administration and at suitable intervals during treatment.

## What to consider

- No ABO or Rh matching is necessary.
- The risk of hepatitis is high; administration is contraindicated in a patient with hepatic disease resulting in fibrinolysis and in a patient with intravascular coagulation who isn't undergoing heparin therapy.

## Managing patients with special needs

# The pediatric patient

## Key facts

- Blood units are prepared in half-unit packs.
- A 22G or 24G catheter is used to administer the blood.
- Usually, 5% to 10% of the total quantity is transfused in the first 15 minutes of therapy; an electronic infusion device must be used to maintain the correct flow rate.
- A child's normal circulating blood volume determines the amount of blood transfused. (The average blood volume for children older than age 1 month is 75 ml/kg; the proportion of blood volume to body weight decreases with age.)

## What to do

- Make sure that informed consent has been obtained.
- Explain the procedure to the child and parent.
- Monitor the child closely, especially during the first 15 minutes of a transfusion, to detect early signs of a reaction.
- Use a blood warmer, if indicated, to prevent hypothermia and cardiac arrhythmias, especially if you're administering blood through a central line.
- Draw blood from a central vein to get more accurate hemoglobin and hematocrit measurements.

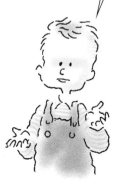

Remember, a plain and simple explanation will help to reassure me.

## What to consider

- In massive hemorrhage and shock, indications for blood component transfusion in children are similar to those for adults.

# The elderly patient

## Key facts

- Age-related slowing of the immune system puts an older adult at risk for delayed transfusion reactions. Because greater quantities of blood products transfuse before signs or symptoms appear, the patient may experience a more severe reaction.
- Elderly patients tend to be less resistant to infection.

## What to do

- Administer half-unit infusions as ordered.
- Be diligent in monitoring the patient for adverse transfusion reactions.

## What to consider

- An elderly patient with preexisting heart disease may be unable to tolerate rapid transfusion of an entire unit of blood without shortness of breath or other signs of heart failure.

# Managing common problems of blood transfusions

## Stopped transfusion

### Key facts

- Possible causes:
  - I.V. container may be too low or empty
  - Blood cells may have settled to bottom of container
  - Flow clamp may be closed

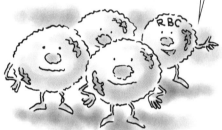

Give us a little nudge so we don't settle on the bottom!

### What to do

- Check that the I.V. container is at least 3′ (1 m) above the level of the I.V. site.
- Make sure that the flow clamp is open.
- Make sure that the blood completely covers the filter; if not, squeeze the drip chamber until it does.
- Gently rock the bag back and forth, agitating blood cells that may have settled on the bottom.
- Untape the dressing over the I.V. site to check the cannula's placement in the vein and reposition if necessary.

### Using a Y-type blood administration set

- Close the flow clamp to the patient, and lower the blood bag.
- Open the normal saline solution line clamp and allow the solution to flow into the blood bag.
- Rehang the blood bag, and open the flow clamp to the patient.
- Reset the flow rate.

# Hematoma

## Key facts

- Bruising at venipuncture site
- Results from bleeding within the tissue at the insertion site

## What to do

- Immediately stop the infusion.
- Remove the needle or catheter.
- Cap the tubing with a new needleless connection.
- Notify the doctor.
- Ice the site for 24 hours; after that, apply warm compresses.
- Promote reabsorption of the hematoma by having the patient gently exercise the affected limb.
- Document your observations and actions.

# Empty blood bag

## Key facts

- A problem when using a Y-type administration set and no replacement blood bag is readily available

## What to do

- When using a Y-type set, take these steps while waiting for the new bag to arrive:
  - Close the blood line clamp.
  - Open the normal saline solution line clamp.
  - Let the normal saline solution run slowly until the new blood arrives.
  - Make sure that you decrease the flow rate or clamp the line before attaching the new unit of blood.

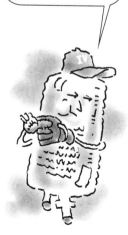

If I've still got some juice—great. If not, you should have my reliever in the bullpen!

## Managing transfusion reactions

## Allergic reaction

### Key facts
- Occurs because of an allergen in the transfused blood
- May progress to an anaphylactic reaction
- Can occur immediately or within 1 hour after infusion
- Severe anaphylactic reactions produce bronchospasm, dyspnea, pulmonary edema, and hypotension

### What to look for
- Chills
- Facial swelling
- Fever
- Hives
- Itching
- Throat swelling
- Wheezing

### What to do
- Stop the blood transfusion immediately.
- Start administering normal saline solution.
- Check and document the patient's vital signs.
- Call the doctor.
- Initiate anaphylaxis protocol.
- Return the remaining blood, a posttransfusion blood sample, and other required samples to the blood bank.

### How to prevent it
- Premedicate the patient with an antihistamine if he has a history of allergic transfusion reactions or if he has had numerous transfusions.
- Observe the patient closely for the first 30 minutes of the transfusion.

# Bacterial contamination reaction

## Key facts

- Usually results from contamination of blood or blood products during the collection process
- Growth of microorganisms increases with increasing storage times and temperature; resulting transfusion reaction commonly related to the endotoxins produced by gram-negative bacteria

## What to look for

- Abdominal cramping
- Chills
- Diarrhea
- Fever
- Kidney failure
- Shock
- Vomiting

## What to do

- Treat the patient with a broad-spectrum antibiotic and a steroid as ordered.

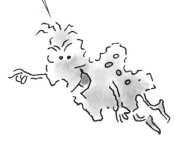

When the crime is bacterial contamination, gram-negative bacteria like me are the usual suspects.

## How to prevent it

- Inspect the blood before the transfusion for gas bubbles, clots, or a dark purple color.
- Use air-free, touch-free methods to draw and deliver blood.
- Maintain strict storage control.
- Change the blood tubing and filter every 4 hours.
- Infuse each unit of blood over 2 to 4 hours; stop the infusion after 4 hours.
- Maintain sterile technique when administering blood products.

# Circulation overload

## Key facts

- May be caused by a blood transfusion (may occur up to 24 hours after completion of the transfusion)
- May result in pulmonary edema
- Elderly patients and patients with heart failure or renal disease at highest risk

## What to look for

- Back pain
- Chest tightness
- Fever and chills
- Flushed feeling
- Headache
- Hypertension
- Increased central venous pressure and jugular vein pressure
- Increased plasma volume

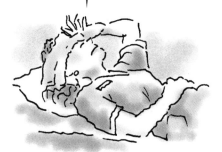

Headache is a key sign of circulation overload (or patient overload in my case!).

## What to do

- Stop the transfusion.
- Maintain the I.V. infusion with normal saline solution.
- Administer oxygen.
- Elevate the patient's head.
- Administer diuretics as ordered.

## How to prevent it

- Transfuse blood slowly.
- Don't transfuse more than 2 units of blood in 4 hours; less for elderly patients, infants, and patients with cardiac conditions.

# Febrile reaction

## Key facts

- Characterized by a temperature increase of 1.8° F (1° C) above the patient's baseline temperature
- Usually results from the patient's anti-HLA antibodies reacting against antigens on the donor's WBCs or platelets
- May occur in approximately 1% of transfusions
- Can occur immediately or within 2 hours after completion of a transfusion

## What to look for

- Chest pain
- Chills
- Dyspnea
- Fever
- Headache
- Hypotension
- Malaise
- Nausea and vomiting
- Nonproductive cough

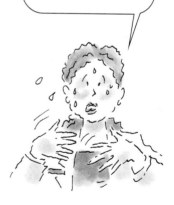

Fever, headache, and nausea can all be signs of a febrile reaction to a blood transfusion (or a really bad day at work).

## What to do

- Relieve symptoms with an antipyretic, antihistamine, or meperidine.
- Use leukocyte-poor or washed RBCs.
- Use a leukocyte removal filter specific to the component.

## How to prevent it

- Premedicate the patient with an antipyretic, an antihistamine and, possibly, a steroid.

# Hemolytic reaction

## Key facts

- Occurs from incompatible blood use or improper storage
- Almost always associated with mislabeling or failing to properly identify the patient
- May progress to shock and renal failure; may be life-threatening

## What to look for

- Bloody oozing at the infusion site
- Burning sensation along the vein receiving the blood
- Chest pain
- Chills and shaking
- Dyspnea
- Facial flushing
- Flank pain
- Hemoglobinuria
- Hypotension
- Oliguria
- Shock

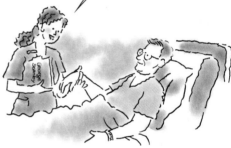

Before we start your I.V., I just want to verify your personal information.

## What to do

- Monitor the patient's blood pressure.
- Treat shock as indicated by the patient's condition, using I.V. fluids, oxygen, epinephrine, a diuretic, and a vasopressor.
- Obtain posttransfusion reaction blood and urine samples.
- Observe for signs of hemorrhage.

## How to prevent it

- Always check the donor and recipient blood types to ensure blood compatibility, and identify the patient with another nurse or a doctor present.
- Transfuse blood slowly for the first 15 to 20 minutes.
- Closely observe the patient for the first 30 minutes.

# Plasma protein incompatibility reaction

## Key facts

- Can be life-threatening
- Usually results from blood that contains immunoglobulin (Ig) A proteins being infused into an IgA-deficient recipient who has developed anti-IgA antibodies
- Usually resembles anaphylaxis

## What to look for

- Abdominal pain
- Cardiac arrest
- Chills
- Dyspnea and wheezing
- Fever
- Flushing and urticaria
- Hypotension
- Shock

## What to do

- Treat the patient for shock by administering oxygen, fluids, epinephrine and, possibly, a steroid, as ordered.

## How to prevent it

- Transfuse only IgA-deficient blood or well-washed RBCs.

# Managing reactions from multiple transfusions

## Bleeding tendencies

### Key facts

- May be caused by a low platelet count, which can develop in stored blood

### What to look for

- Abnormal bleeding
- Abnormal clotting values
- Oozing from a cut or break in the skin surface

### What to do

- Administer platelets.
- Monitor the platelet count.

### How to prevent it

- Use only fresh blood (less than 7 days old) when possible.

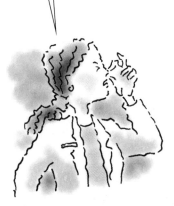

Keep it fresh! Using blood that's less than 7 days old is the best way to prevent bleeding problems from multiple transfusions.

# Elevated blood ammonia level

## Key facts
- Possibly caused by transfusions of stored blood

## What to look for
- Confusion
- Forgetfulness
- Elevated ammonia levels
- Sweet mouth odor

## What to do
- Monitor the patient's ammonia level.
- Decrease the amount of protein in the patient's diet.
- If indicated, administer neomycin or lactulose.

## How to prevent it
- Use only RBCs, FFP, or fresh blood, especially if the patient has hepatic disease.

# Hemosiderosis

## Key facts
- Accumulation of an iron-containing pigment (hemosiderin), possibly associated with RBC destruction in patients who receive many transfusions

## What to look for
- Iron plasma level greater than 200 mg/dl

## What to do
- Perform a phlebotomy to remove the excess iron.

## How to prevent it
- Administer blood only when absolutely necessary.

# Hypocalcemia

## Key facts

- May be caused by citrate (a drug used to preserve blood) toxicity if the blood is infused too rapidly (because citrate binds with calcium)
- May follow normal citrate metabolism that's hindered by a liver disorder

## What to look for

- Cardiac arrhythmias
- Hypotension
- Muscle cramps
- Nausea
- Seizures
- Tingling in the fingers
- Vomiting

## What to do

- Monitor the patient's potassium and calcium levels.
- Slow or stop the transfusion, depending on the patient's reaction.
- Prepare for a more severe reaction in a hypothermic patient or a patient with an elevated potassium level.
- Slowly administer calcium gluconate I.V.

## How to prevent it

- Use blood less than 2 days old if administering multiple units.
- Infuse blood slowly.

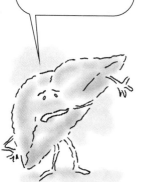

A disorder in my neck of the woods can hinder citrate metabolism.

# Hypothermia

## Key facts
- Can be caused by a rapid infusion of large amounts of cold blood

## What to look for
- Cardiac arrhythmias, which may become life-threatening
- Hypotension
- Shaking chills
- Cardiac arrest—possible if the patient's core temperature falls below 86° F (30° C).

## What to do
- Stop the transfusion.
- Warm the patient with blankets.
- Obtain an electrocardiogram (ECG).

## How to prevent it
- Warm blood to 95° to 98° F (35° to 36.7° C), especially before massive transfusions (transfusing the patient's total blood volume in less than 24 hours).

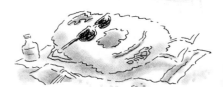

Ahhh. A day at the beach...just what the doctor ordered!

# Increased oxygen affinity for hemoglobin

## Key facts

- A blood transfusion can cause a decreased level of 2,3-diphosphoglycerate (2,3-DPG), which affects the oxyhemoglobin dissociation curve—representative of hemoglobin saturation and desaturation in graph form.
- Levels of 2,3-DPG (as well as other factors) cause the curve to shift either to the right (causing a decrease in oxygen affinity) or to the left (causing an increase in oxygen affinity).
- Low 2,3-DPG levels produce a shift to the left, causing an increase in oxygen affinity for hemoglobin; oxygen stays in the bloodstream and isn't released into other tissues.

## What to look for

- Depressed respiratory rate, especially in patients with chronic lung disease

## What to do

- Monitor arterial blood gas levels, and give respiratory support as needed.

## How to prevent it

- Use only RBCs or fresh blood if possible.

# Potassium intoxication

## Key facts

- Most commonly occurs in transfusions of more than 2 units of blood because some cells in stored RBCs may leak potassium into the plasma

## What to look for

- Bradycardia that may proceed to cardiac arrest
- Diarrhea
- ECG changes with tall, peaked T waves
- Intestinal colic
- Irritability
- Muscle weakness
- Oliguria
- Renal failure

## What to do

- Obtain an ECG.
- Administer sodium polystyrene sulfonate (Kayexalate) orally or by enema.

## How to prevent it

- Use fresh blood when transfusing the patient's total blood volume in less than 24 hours.

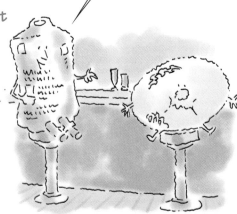

You OK, buddy? Better go easy on the potassium plasma punch. I'm tellin' ya, that stuff really packs a wallop.

# Chemotherapy infusions

# 6

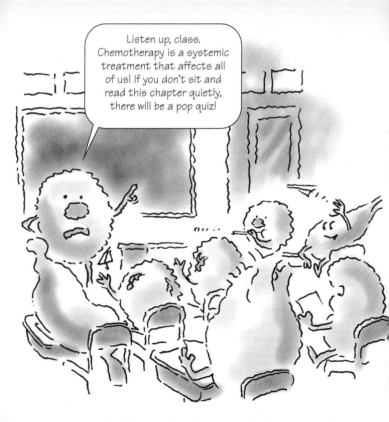

## Understanding I.V. chemotherapy

- Unlike surgery and radiation, which target a specific tumor site, chemotherapy works throughout the entire body to eradicate disease or cancerous growth.
- Chemotherapy involves administration of repeated doses of one or more drugs to kill cancerous cells (a single course of chemotherapy typically involves repeating doses of a drug on a cyclic basis).
  - Each cycle can be repeated daily, weekly, biweekly, or every 3 to 4 weeks.
  - Cycles are carefully planned so normal cells can regenerate; timing depends on the cycle of the targeted cells and the return of normal blood counts.
  - Usually, no benefits are seen until after three treatment cycles, but response time varies; some patients don't respond.

# Chemotherapeutic drugs

## Key facts

- Healthy and cancerous cells pass through similar life cycles and are similarly vulnerable to chemotherapeutic drugs.
- Chemotherapeutic drugs are categorized according to their pharmacologic action and the way they interfere with cell production.
- Treatment with cycle-specific versus cycle-nonspecific chemotherapeutic drugs depends on a combination of patient factors (age, overall condition, allergies, sensitivities) and disease factors (tumor type, cancer stage).

### Cycle-specific drugs

- Designed to disrupt a specific biochemical process, making them effective only during specific phases of the cell cycle
- Divided into three categories: antimetabolites, enzymes, and plant alkaloids

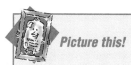

*Picture this!*

# The cell cycle and chemotherapeutic drugs

All cells cycle through five phases. Chemotherapeutic drugs that are active on cells during one or more of these phases are called *cycle-specific*. This illustration shows what happens at each phase of the cell cycle and gives examples of cycle-specific drugs that are active during each phase.

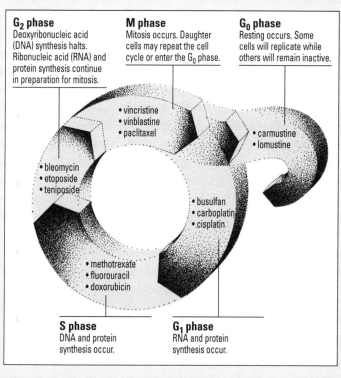

**$G_2$ phase**
Deoxyribonucleic acid (DNA) synthesis halts. Ribonucleic acid (RNA) and protein synthesis continue in preparation for mitosis.

**M phase**
Mitosis occurs. Daughter cells may repeat the cell cycle or enter the $G_0$ phase.

**$G_0$ phase**
Resting occurs. Some cells will replicate while others will remain inactive.

- vincristine
- vinblastine
- paclitaxel

- carmustine
- lomustine

- bleomycin
- etoposide
- teniposide

- busulfan
- carboplatin
- cisplatin

- methotrexate
- fluorouracil
- doxorubicin

**S phase**
DNA and protein synthesis occur.

**$G_1$ phase**
RNA and protein synthesis occur.

- When administered, cells in the resting phase survive

## Cycle-nonspecific drugs

- Prolonged action is independent of the cell cycle, allowing the drugs to act on reproducing and resting cells
- Divided into five categories: alkylating agents, antibiotic antineoplastics, antineoplastics, miscellaneous, and nitrosoureas
- During single administration, a fixed percentage of normal and malignant cells die

## Other drugs

- Work in the intracellular environment
- Include steroids, hormones, and antihormones:

– *Steroids* make malignant cells vulnerable to damage from cell-specific drugs.

– *Hormones* alter the environment of cells by affecting the permeability of their membranes.

– *Antihormones* affect hormone-dependent tumors by binding to the hormone receptors and inhibiting hormone-mediated growth in the tumor tissue.

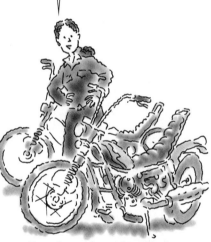

Well, I've narrowed it down to these two — the Biochemical Process Disruptor, with the cell-specific timing action...and the Independent Terminator, with the nonspecific piston-firing mechanism.

# Comparing chemotherapeutic drugs

| Category | Characteristics | Toxic effects |
|---|---|---|
| **Cycle-specific** | | |
| *Antimetabolites* cytarabine, floxuridine, fluorouracil, hydroxyurea, methotrexate, thioguanine | • Interfere with nucleic acid synthesis<br>• Attack during S phase of cell cycle | • Effects on bone marrow (myelosuppression), central nervous system (CNS), and GI system |
| *Enzymes* asparaginase | • Useful only for leukemias | • Hypersensitivity reactions |
| *Plant alkaloids* vinblastine, vincristine | • Cycle-specific to M phase<br>• Prevent mitotic spindle formation | • Effects on CNS and GI system<br>• Myelosuppression<br>• Tissue damage |
| **Cycle-nonspecific** | | |
| *Alkylating agents* carboplatin, cisplatin, cyclophosphamide, ifosfamide, thiotepa | • Disrupt DNA replication | • Infertility<br>• Secondary carcinoma<br>• Effects on renal system |
| *Antibiotics* bleomycin, doxorubicin, idarubicin, mitomycin, mitoxantrone | • Bind with DNA to inhibit synthesis of DNA and RNA | • Effects on GI, renal, and hepatic systems<br>• Effects on bone marrow |

*(continued)*

## Comparing chemotherapeutic drugs *(continued)*

| Category | Characteristics | Toxic effects |
|---|---|---|
| ***Cytoprotective agents*** | | |
| dexrazoxane, mesna | • Protect normal tissue by binding with metabolites of other cytotoxic drugs | • None |
| ***Folic acid analogs*** | | |
| leucovorin | • Antidote for methotrexate toxicity | • Hypersensitivity reaction possible |
| ***Hormone and hormone inhibitors*** | | |
| androgens (testolactone), antiandrogens (flutamide), antiestrogens (tamoxifen), estrogens (estramustine), gonadotropin (leuprolide), progestins (megestrol) | • Interfere with binding of normal hormones to receptor proteins<br>• Manipulate hormone levels<br>• Alter hormone environment<br>• Mechanism of action not always clear<br>• Usually palliative, not curative | • No known toxic effect |

# Chemotherapy protocols

## Key facts

- Involves giving drugs in a specific order and combination to maximize therapeutic effect
- More cancerous cells destroyed by combining chemotherapeutic drugs because the drug attacks the cancer cell at different points in the cell cycle
- Fewer adverse effects with combination therapy
- Chemotherapy combinations individualized for the patient and the type of cancer
- Generic or trade names may be used in protocols; when a trade name is used, the generic name will be in parentheses

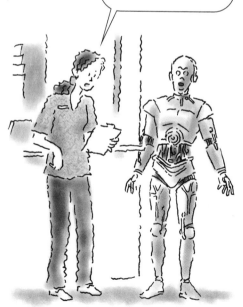

## Sample chemotherapy protocols

Chemotherapy drugs are commonly given in combinations called *protocols*.

| Specific cancers | Protocols | Drugs |
| --- | --- | --- |
| Acute lymphocytic leukemia, induction | DVP | • daunorubicin<br>• vincristine<br>• prednisone |
| Bladder cancer | CISCA | • cisplatin<br>• cyclophosphamide<br>• Adriamycin (doxorubicin) |
| Breast cancer | AC | • Adriamycin (doxorubicin)<br>• cyclophosphamide |
| Cervical cancer | MOBP | • mitomycin<br>• Oncovin (vincristine)<br>• bleomycin<br>• Platinol (cisplatin) |
| Lung cancer, small-cell | CAE (ACE) | • cyclophosphamide<br>• Adriamycin (doxorubicin)<br>• etoposide |
| Lymphoma (non-Hodgkin's) | CVP (COP) | • cyclophosphamide<br>• Oncovin (vincristine)<br>• prednisone |
| Lymphoma (Hodgkin's disease) | ABVD | • Adriamycin (doxorubicin)<br>• bleomycin<br>• vinblastine<br>• dacarbazine |

# Understanding immunotherapy

- Involves the use of natural substances, normally found in small amounts in the body, which have been developed scientifically to treat cancer and other diseases (rheumatoid arthritis, hepatitis C)
- Mainly includes administration of biological response modifiers and the use of immunotherapy

## Biological response modifiers

- Work by altering the body's response to therapy
- May cause direct cytotoxicity
- Includes monoclonal antibodies, cytokines (interferons, interleukins), colony-stimulating factors, and vaccines

## Immunotherapy

- Uses drugs to enhance the body's natural ability to destroy cancer cells
- Promotes effective immune response to tumors by altering the way cells grow, mature, and respond to cancer cells
- May include administration of monoclonal antibodies and immunomodulatory cytokines

## Targeting tumors with monoclonal antibodies

A more recent form of biotherapy, monoclonal antibodies are mass-produced in the laboratory from a single clone that recognizes only a single unique antigen. They specifically target tumor cells, manipulating the body's natural resources instead of introducing toxic substances that aren't selective and can't differentiate between normal and abnormal processes or cells.

| Drug | Treatment |
|------|-----------|
| Rituximab | • Specifically indicated for relapsed or refractory low-grade Hodgkin's disease and non-Hodgkin's lymphoma |
| Herceptin | • Beneficial against metastatic breast cancer<br>• May be used as a first-line treatment in combination with chemotherapy or as a second-line single agent |

# Immunomodulatory cytokines: Infection-fighting messengers

These intracellular messenger proteins (proteins that deliver messages within cells) are naturally occurring substances that are injected into the body to help fight infection in cancer patients.

## Colony-stimulating factors
• Substances naturally produced by the body that stimulate the growth of different cell types found in the blood and the immune system
• Have been helpful in the care of patients receiving myelosuppressive therapy

### Erythropoietin
• Induces erythroid maturation (maturation of red blood cells [RBCs]) and increases the release of reticulocytes from the bone marrow, which stimulates the production of RBCs, possibly reducing the number of blood transfusions needed by the patient

### Granulocyte colony-stimulating factor
• Stimulates proliferation, differentiation, and functional activity of neutrophils, causing a rapid rise in white blood cell count

• Given to reduce the incidence of infection in patients receiving chemotherapeutic drugs

### Granulocyte-macrophage colony-stimulating factor
• Indicated for older patients receiving chemotherapy for acute myelogenous leukemia, for patients undergoing bone marrow transplantation, and for peripheral blood progenitor collection

## Interferon
• Approved for treating chronic myeloid leukemia, hairy cell leukemia, and acquired immunodeficiency syndrome–related Kaposi's sarcoma
• Used with low-grade malignant lymphoma, multiple myeloma, and renal cell carcinoma

## Interleukins
• Cytokines that primarily function to deliver messages to leukocytes
• Interleukin-2 — an approved anticancer agent that stimulates the proliferation and cytolytic activity of T cells and natural killer cells; high doses effective in a few patients with metastatic renal cell carcinoma and melanoma

*(continued)*

**Immunomodulatory cytokines: Infection-fighting messengers**
*(continued)*

• Other interleukins under investigation for cancer therapy

**Tumor necrosis factor**
• Plays a role in inflammatory response to tumors and cancer cells

• Has produced impressive antitumor responses in animal studies
• Considered investigational

## Preparing to administer I.V. chemotherapy

## Gathering the equipment

Gather together all necessary equipment:
- patient's medication order or record
- prescribed drugs
- appropriate diluent (if necessary)
- medication labels
- long-sleeved gown, chemotherapy gloves, and face shield or goggles and face mask
- I.V. access supplies (if necessary)
- sterile normal saline solution
- 20G needles
- hydrophobic filter or dispensing pin
- syringes with luer-lock fittings and needles of various sizes
- I.V. tubing with luer-lock fittings
- 70% alcohol
- sterile gauze pads
- plastic bags with "hazardous drug" labels
- sharps disposal container and leakproof hazardous waste container
- chemotherapy spill kit
- extravasation kit.

## Organizing drug preparation areas

*What to do*

- Prepare chemotherapeutic drugs in a well-ventilated work-space.
- Perform all drug admixing or compounding within a Class II Biological Safety Cabinet or a "vertical" laminar airflow hood with a HEPA filter (vented to the outside). The hood pulls the aerosolized chemotherapeutic drug particles away from the compounder. If a Class II Biological Safety Cabinet isn't available, the Occupational Safety and Health Administration (OSHA) recommends that you wear a special respirator.
- Ensure easy access to a sink, alcohol pads, and gauze pads.
- Ensure easy access to OSHA-required chemotherapy hazardous waste containers (puncture-, shatter-, and leakproof), sharps containers, and chemotherapy spill kits (make sure red sharps containers are available for disposal of all contaminated sharps such as needles).
- Gather yellow biohazard labels for labeling all chemotherapy-contaminated I.V. bags, tubing, filters, and syringes.

## Understanding chemotherapy safety precautions

## Wearing protective clothing

### Key facts

- Essential protective gear includes a cuffed gown, gloves, and a face shield or goggles and a face mask.

### What to do

- Wear disposable gowns that are water-resistant and lint-free, and have long sleeves, knitted cuffs, and a closed front.
- Wear disposable, powder-free gloves (powder can carry contamination from the drugs into the surrounding air) made of thick latex or thick nonlatex material.
- Use double-gloving when available gloves aren't of the best quality.

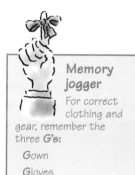

**Memory jogger**

For correct clothing and gear, remember the three G's:

Gown

Gloves

Goggles.

# Taking general safety measures

## Key facts

- At the local level, most health care facilities require nurses and pharmacists involved in the preparation and delivery of chemotherapeutic drugs to complete a certification program, covering the safe delivery of chemotherapeutic drugs and care of the patient with cancer.

## What to do

- Take care to protect staff, patients, and the environment from unnecessary exposure to chemotherapeutic drugs.
- Make sure your facility's protocols for spills are available in all areas where chemotherapeutic drugs are handled, including patient-care areas.
- Refrain from eating, drinking, smoking, or applying cosmetics in the drug-preparation area.

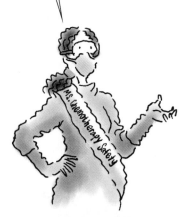

I'd like to thank my training and my facility's protocols for giving me the opportunity to share this gift of safety with my patients and my coworkers.

# Preparing drugs safely

*What to do*

- Put on protective gear before you begin to compound the chemotherapeutic drugs.
- Before preparing the drugs, clean the work area with 70% alcohol and a disposable towel; do the same after you're finished and after a spill.
- Discard towels used to clean the preparation area into the yellow leakproof chemotherapy waste container.
- Use aseptic technique when preparing all drugs.
- Use blunt-ended needles whenever possible.
- Change gloves whenever a tear or puncture occurs.
- Wash your hands before putting on and after removing gloves.
- Use needles with a hydrophobic filter to remove solutions from vials.
- Vent vials with a hydrophobic filter or use the negative pressure technique to reduce the amount of aerosolized drugs.
- When you break ampules, wrap a gauze pad around the neck of the vial to reduce the risk of droplet contamination and glove puncture.
- Wear a face shield or face mask and goggles to protect yourself against splashes and aerosolized drugs.

# Disposal and exposure

## What to do

### Disposal of waste

- Place all contaminated needles in the sharps container; don't recap needles.
- Use only syringes and I.V. sets that have a luer-lock fitting.
- Label all chemotherapeutic drugs with a yellow biohazard label.
- Transport the prepared chemotherapeutic drugs in a sealable plastic bag that's prominently labeled with a yellow chemotherapy biohazard label.
- Don't leave the drug-preparation area while wearing the protective gear you wore during drug preparation.

### Dealing with accidental exposure

- If a chemotherapeutic drug comes in contact with your skin, wash the area thoroughly with soap and water to prevent drug absorption into the skin.
- If the drug comes in contact with your eye, immediately flush the eye with water or isotonic eyewash for at least 5 minutes, while holding the eyelid open.
- After an accidental exposure, notify your supervisor immediately.

# Handling a chemotherapy spill

## What to do

- Follow your facility's protocol (probably based on OSHA guidelines).
- Put on protective garments if you aren't already wearing them.
- Isolate the area and contain the spill with absorbent materials from a chemotherapy spill kit.
- Use the disposable dustpan and scraper to collect broken glass or desiccant absorbing powder.
- Carefully place the dustpan, scraper, and collected spill in a leakproof, puncture-proof, chemotherapy-designated hazardous waste container.
- Prevent aerosolization of the drug at all times.
- Clean the spill area with a detergent or bleach solution.
- Per your facility's policy, notify the necessary individuals regarding the spill.

---

### Inside a chemotherapy spill kit

A chemotherapy spill kit should contain:
- long-sleeved gown that's water-resistant and nonpermeable, with cuffs and back closure
- shoe covers
- two pairs of powder-free surgical gloves (for double gloving)
- respirator mask
- chemical splash goggles
- disposable dustpan and plastic scraper (for collecting broken glass)
- plastic-backed absorbent towels or spill-control pillows
- desiccant powder or granules (for absorbing wet contents)
- disposable sponges
- two large cytotoxic waste disposal bags.

# Administering chemotherapeutic drugs

- Each treatment cycle may involve infusion of one or more medications, depending on the specific cancer or disease.
- Treatment timing and doses are adjusted to maximize drug effects against cancer cells while allowing time for normal cells to recover between courses.
- Chemotherapeutic drugs are classified as vesicants, nonvesicants, and irritants, according to their potential for tissue damage.
- Safe administration of chemotherapeutic drugs depends on knowledge of potential tissue damage and careful monitoring for complications.

## Tissue damage risk

**Vesicants**
Vesicants cause a reaction so severe that blisters form and tissue is damaged or destroyed.

Chemotherapeutic vesicants include:
- dactinomycin
- daunorubicin
- doxorubicin
- idarubicin
- mechlorethamine
- mitomycin
- mitoxantrone
- nitrogen mustard
- vinblastine
- vincristine
- vinorelbine.

**Nonvesicants**
Nonvesicants don't cause irritation or damage.

Chemotherapeutic nonvesicants include:
- asparaginase
- bleomycin
- carboplatin
- cyclophosphamide
- cytarabine
- floxuridine
- fluorouracil
- ifosfamide.

**Irritants**
Irritants can cause a local venous response, with or without a skin reaction.

Chemotherapeutic irritants include:
- dacarbazine
- streptozocin.

# Performing a preadministration check

## Key facts
- Performed as a safety measure

## What to do
- Double-check the order with another chemotherapy-certified nurse.
- Check the patient's blood count. Depending on your facility's policy, notify the doctor for approval if the patient's blood count drops below a predetermined level.
- Check the route of the drug.
- Check if the drug is a vesicant or an irritant and which should be administered first or last.
- Confirm written orders for antiemetics, fluids, diuretics, or electrolyte supplements.

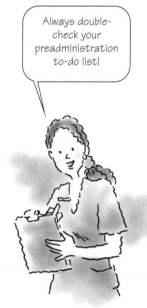

Always double-check your preadministration to-do list!

# Administering a vesicant

## Key facts

- These drugs can cause severe blistering and tissue damage (from extravasation), requiring careful administration and monitoring.
- When giving through a peripheral vein, use a low-pressure infusion pump.
- When giving a continuous infusion, use a central venous catheter.

## What to do

- Make sure the extravasation kit is readily available.
- Make sure the chemotherapy spill kit is available.
- Use a distal vein that allows successive proximal venipunctures.
- Avoid using the hand, antecubital space, damaged areas, or areas of compromised circulation.
- Don't probe or "fish" for veins.

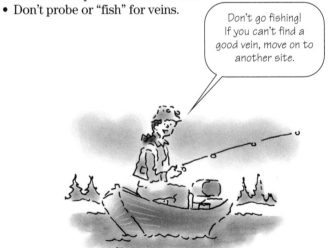

Don't go fishing! If you can't find a good vein, move on to another site.

- Place a transparent dressing over the site.
- Start the push delivery or infusion with normal saline solution.
- Inspect the site for swelling or erythema.
- Tell the patient to report any burning, stinging, pain, pruritus, or temperature changes near the site (which may signal extravasation of the vesicant solution into surrounding tissue — an emergency requiring immediate attention).
- If extravasation occurs, stop the infusion immediately and follow your facility's policy for treatment; also notify the doctor.
- Following administration, flush the line with 20 ml of normal saline solution.

# Administering nonvesicant or irritant drugs

## Key facts

- Nonvesicants may infiltrate into surrounding tissue at the infusion site, requiring careful monitoring during administration.
- Irritants may cause vein flaring, phlebitis, or thrombosis and require careful monitoring.

## What to do

### During administration

- Check for infiltration.
- If you note swelling at the I.V. insertion site, the solution is infiltrating and the I.V. should be stopped and the needle removed.
- Observe around the site for streaky redness along the vein and other skin changes.
- Tell the patient to report burning, stinging, or pain at or near the site.
- Listen to what the patient has to say about his level of comfort; sudden discomfort during administration or flushing could indicate infiltration.

### After administration

- Dispose of all used needles and contaminated sharps in the red sharps container.
- Dispose of personal protective gear, glasses, and gloves in the yellow chemotherapeutic waste container.
- Dispose of unused medications (considered hazardous waste) according to your facility's policy.
- Wash your hands thoroughly with soap and water, even though you've worn gloves.
- Remember to wear protective clothing when handling the patient's body fluids for 48 hours after chemotherapy treatment has ended, following your facility's policy and procedures.

- Document the sequence in which the drugs were administered.
- Document the site accessed, the gauge and length of the catheter, and the number of attempts.
- Document the name, dose, and route of the administered drugs.
- Document the type and volume of the I.V. solutions and adverse reactions and nursing interventions.

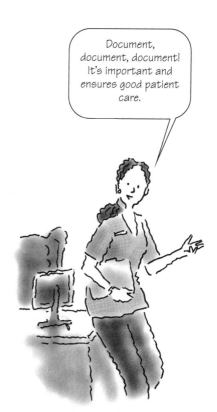

Document, document, document! It's important and ensures good patient care.

# Managing complications

- Because of the powerful systemic effects of chemotherapeutic drugs, complications can occur in every organ system.
- Complications are categorized according to where or when exposure to the drug began:
  - infusion-site related
  - hypersensitivity or anaphylactic reactions
  - short-term
  - long-term.
- Educating patients about potential adverse effects (and treatment options) beforehand may help lessen the emotional trauma when adverse effects occur.

# Alopecia

## Key facts

- Hair loss that occurs as chemotherapeutic drugs destroy the rapidly growing cells of hair follicles
- May be minimal or severe depending on the type of drug, dose and length of treatment, and the patient's reaction
- Usually begins to occur within 2 to 3 weeks after treatment starts
- Almost always short-term

## What to look for

- Hair loss that may include eyebrows, lashes, and body hair.

## What to do

- Prepare the patient for the possibility of hair loss, why it occurs, and how much to expect.
- Give the patient time to decide whether to order a wig; provide a list of reputable manufacturers and organizations.
- Emphasize the need for head protection from sunburn and heat loss in the winter.
- Inform the patient that new hair may be a different texture or color.
- Inform the patient that his scalp will become sore at times due to the follicles swelling.

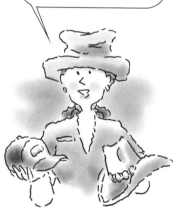

To women, hair loss can be the most devastating adverse effect of chemotherapy. Help them anyway you can!

## How to prevent it

- For patients with long hair, suggest cutting it shorter before treatment because washing and brushing cause more hair loss.

# Anemia

## Key facts

- Occurs as chemotherapeutic drugs destroy healthy cells and cancer cells
- Involves destruction of red blood cells (RBCs) that can't be replaced by the bone marrow
- Long-term complication of chemotherapy

## What to look for

- Dizziness, fatigue, pallor, and shortness of breath after minimal exertion
- Low hemoglobin and hematocrit
- May develop slowly over several courses of treatment

## What to do

- Monitor hemoglobin level and RBC count; report dropping values.
- Monitor hematocrit (dehydration from nausea, vomiting, and anorexia will cause hemoconcentration, yielding falsely high readings); report dropping values.
- Be prepared to administer a blood transfusion or erythropoietin.

## How to prevent it

- Instruct the patient to rest frequently, increase his intake of iron-rich foods, and take a multivitamin with iron as prescribed.
- If the patient has been prescribed a drug such as epoetin, make sure he understands how to take the drug (including adverse effects to watch for and report).

# Diarrhea

## Key facts

- Occurs because the rapidly dividing cells of the intestinal mucosa are killed
- May produce weight loss, fluid and electrolyte imbalance, and malnutrition
- Short-term complication

## What to look for

- An increase in the volume of stool compared with the patient's normal bowel habits

## What to do

- Assess frequency, color, and consistency of stool.
- Encourage the patient to drink plenty of fluids, and give I.V. fluids and potassium supplements as ordered.
- Adjust the patient's diet as ordered.
- Provide good perianal skin care.

## How to prevent it

- Administer antidiarrheal medications as ordered.

# Extravasation

## Key facts

- Inadvertent leakage of a vesicant solution into surrounding tissue
- An emergency situation that requires immediate treatment
- Infusion-site related

## What to look for

- Initially, may resemble signs and symptoms of infiltration
- Possible symptom progression: blisters; skin, muscle, tissue, and fat necrosis; tissue sloughing
- Possible damage to outer surface of veins, arteries, and nerves

## What to do

- Remove the I.V. catheter if you suspect extravasation.
- If a vesicant has extravasated, quickly take these emergency steps to limit the damage:
  – Stop the infusion and notify the doctor.
  – Check your facility's policy to determine if the I.V. catheter is to be removed or left in place to infuse corticosteroids or a specific antidote.
  – Instill the appropriate antidote (follow your facility's policy). Give the antidote by instilling it through the existing I.V. catheter or by using a 1-ml syringe to inject small amounts subcutaneously in a circle around the extravasated area.
  – After the antidote is injected, remove the I.V. catheter.

## How to prevent it

- Verify I.V. line patency and placement by flushing with normal saline solution and observing the site for swelling (blood return is inconclusive and shouldn't be used to determine if the I.V. catheter is correctly seated in the peripheral vein).
- Use a transparent, semipermeable dressing for site inspection.
- When in doubt, take out the line.

# Hypersensitivity or anaphylactic reactions

## Key facts
- Can occur with giving the initial dose of a drug, or during subsequent infusions of the same drug
- Can occur at the beginning, middle, or end of the infusion
- Hypersensitivity risk varies according to drug given

### Hypersensitivity risks

**High risk**
- Asparaginase
- Paclitaxel
- Rituximab

**Moderate to low risk**
- Anthracyclines
- Bleomycin
- Carboplatin
- Cisplatin
- Cyclosporine
- Etoposide
- Melphalan
- Methotrexate
- Procarbazine
- Teniposide

**Very low risk**
- Chlorambucil
- Cyclophosphamide
- Cytarabine
- Dacarbazine
- Fluorouracil
- Ifosfamide
- Mitoxantrone

## What to look for
- Specific signs and symptoms vary with the severity of the reaction.
- Severe hypersensitivity and anaphylaxis reactions are considered emergencies and require immediate treatment.

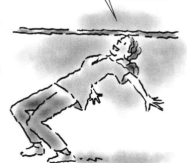

How low can your hypersensitivity risk go?

## Signs and symptoms of immediate hypersensitivity

An immediate hypersensitivity reaction to a chemotherapeutic drug will appear within 5 minutes after starting the drug.

| Organ system | Subjective complaints | Objective findings |
|---|---|---|
| *Respiratory* | Dyspnea, inability to speak, tightness in chest | Stridor, bronchospasm, decreased air movement |
| *Skin* | Pruritus, urticaria | Cyanosis, urticaria, angioedema, cold and clammy skin |
| *Cardiovascular* | Chest pain, increased heart rate | Tachycardia, hypotension, arrhythmias |
| *Central nervous system* | Dizziness, agitation, anxiety | Decreased sensorium, loss of consciousness |

## What to do

Treatment depends the severity of the reaction, and usually involves these steps:

- Stop the infusion.
- Begin a rapid infusion of normal saline solution to quickly dilute the drug.
- Check the patient's vital signs.
- Notify the doctor.
- Administer emergency drugs as ordered:
  - Antihistamines are typically given first, followed by corticosteroids and bronchodilators.
  - Epinephrine is given first in severe anaphylactic reactions.

- After you've administered the drug, monitor the patient's vital signs and pulse oximetry every 5 minutes until he's stable, and then every 15 minutes for 1 to 2 hours — or follow your facility's policies and procedures for treatment of acute allergic reactions.
- Throughout the episode, maintain the patient's airway, oxygenation, and tissue perfusion.
- Make sure life-support equipment is available in case the patient fails to respond.
- Reassure the patient and his family; such reactions can be very frightening.

## How to prevent it

- If hypersensitivity is known, may premedicate with an antihistamine and a corticosteroid

**Memory jogger**

When your patient has an immediate hypersensitivity reaction, let these three pairs of words guide your response:

- **S**top & **s**tay (stop the infusion and stay with the patient)
- **C**heck & **c**all (check vital signs and call the doctor)
- **O**pen & **o**rdered (open the I.V. line containing normal saline solution and administer ordered medications).

# Leukopenia

## Key facts

- Reduced leukocytes or white blood cells (WBCs)
- Occurs as WBCs and cancer cells are destroyed by the chemotherapeutic drugs
- Long-term complication

## What to look for

- Susceptibility to infections
- Neutropenia (an absolute neutrophil count less than 1,500 cells/μl)

## What to do

- Watch for the nadir (the point of lowest blood cell count, usually 7 to 14 days after the last treatment).
- Be prepared to administer colony-stimulating factors.
- Institute neutropenic precautions in the hospitalized patient.
- Teach the patient and caregiver about:
  – good hygiene practices
  – signs and symptoms of infection
  – the importance of checking the patient's temperature regularly
  – how to prepare a low-microbe diet
  – how to care for vascular access devices.
- Instruct the patient to avoid:
  – crowds
  – people with respiratory infections
  – fresh fruit
  – fresh flowers
  – plants.

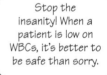

Stop the insanity! When a patient is low on WBCs, it's better to be safe than sorry.

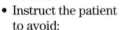

# Nausea and vomiting

## Key facts

- Can occur according to three different patterns:
  - anticipatory
  - acute
  - delayed
- Short-term complication
- Prevention and treatment depend on the specific type of nausea and vomiting

### Anticipatory nausea and vomiting

- Nausea and vomiting that's a learned response from previous nausea and vomiting after a dose of chemotherapy
- Associated with high anxiety levels (act as a trigger)

### Acute nausea and vomiting

- Nausea or vomiting occurring within the first 24 hours of treatment (depends on the emetogenic [vomit-inducing] potential of the drug and on the combination of drugs, doses, rates of administration, and patient characteristics)

### Delayed nausea and vomiting

- Nausea or vomiting starting or continuing beyond 24 hours after chemotherapy has begun

## What to do

### Anticipatory nausea and vomiting

- Administer posttreatment control of nausea and vomiting, which may prevent future anticipatory episodes.

### Acute nausea and vomiting

- Treat with antiemetic drugs, including dexamethasone, granisetron, lorazepam, metoclopramide, ondansetron, prochlorperazine.

### Delayed nausea and vomiting
- Treat with ordered medication; serotonin antagonists, corticosteroids, various antihistamines, benzodiazepines, and metoclopramide are usually effective.

## How to prevent it

### Anticipatory nausea and vomiting
- Have the patient take lorazepam at least 1 hour before arriving for treatment.
- Patients with overwhelming anxiety may need I.V. lorazepam before chemotherapy is administered.

### Acute nausea and vomiting
- Before chemotherapy begins, administer an antiemetic to reduce severity of symptoms.
- Treat with ordered medication; serotonin antagonists, corticosteroids, various antihistamines, benzodiazepines, and metoclopramide are usually effective.

### Delayed nausea and vomiting
- Administer an antiemetic before chemotherapy begins.
- In some patients, treat with an antiemetic for 3 days or longer after chemotherapy treatment.

# Stomatitis

## Key facts

- Inflammation of the lining of the oral mucosa
- Can spread into the esophagus (esophagitis) and pharynx (pharyngitis)
- Can lead to fluid and electrolyte imbalance and malnutrition if the patient can't chew or swallow adequate food or fluid
- Short-term complication

## What to look for

- Painful mouth ulcers that range from mild to severe appearing 3 to 7 days after certain chemotherapeutic drugs are given

## What to do

- Instruct the patient to perform meticulous oral hygiene.
- Administer topical anesthetic mixtures as appropriate.
- If pain is severe, administer opioid analgesics, as ordered, until the ulcers heal.

## How to prevent it

- Instruct the patient to suck on ice chips while receiving certain drugs that cause stomatitis; this decreases the blood supply to the mouth, thus decreasing ulcer formation.

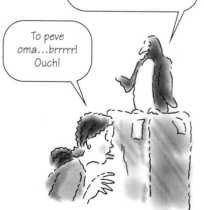

If she weren't so tongue-tied, she'd tell you that sucking on ice chips while taking drugs that cause stomatitis can decrease ulcer formation.

To peve oma...brrrrr! Ouch!

# Thrombocytopenia

## Key facts
- Reduced blood cell platelet count caused by chemotherapeutic drugs
- Long-term complication

## What to look for
- Bleeding gums
- Coffee-ground emesis
- Hematuria
- Hypermenorrhea
- Increased bruising
- Petechiae
- Tarry stool

## What to do
- Monitor the patient's platelet count:
  – less than 50,000 cells/µl means a moderate risk of excessive bleeding
  – less than 20,000 cells/µl means a major risk and the patient may need a platelet transfusion.
- Avoid unnecessary I.M. injections or venipunctures; when necessary, apply pressure for at least 5 minutes, followed by a pressure dressing.
- Instruct the patient to:
  – take necessary precautions to avoid cuts and bruises
  – shave with an electric razor
  – avoid blowing his nose
  – stay away from irritants that could trigger sneezing
  – avoid using rectal thermometers.
- Instruct the patient to report sudden headaches (which could indicate potentially fatal intracranial bleeding).

# Parenteral nutrition

# 7

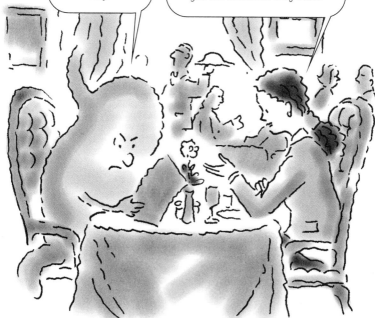

## Understanding nutritional deficiencies

- Most deficiencies involve insufficient protein and calories.
- Protein-energy malnutrition is also called *protein-calorie malnutrition*.

### What causes it

- Nonfunctional GI tract
- Decreased food intake due to illness, decreased physical ability, injury, surgery, sepsis, or GI disorders such as paralytic ileus
- Increased metabolic needs due to fever, burns, trauma, disease, or stress
- Combination of these factors

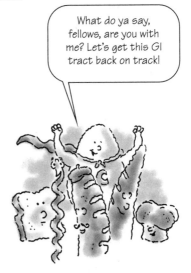

What do ya say, fellows, are you with me? Let's get this GI tract back on track!

# Effects of protein-calorie deficiencies

## Key facts

- When the body detects a protein-calorie deficiency, it draws reserve energy from three sources: glycogen, fats stored in adipose tissue, and essential visceral and somatic body proteins.

  – First, the body mobilizes and converts glycogen to glucose (glycogenolysis).

  – If necessary, the body draws energy from the fats stored in adipose tissue.

  – As a last resort, the body taps its store of essential visceral proteins (serum albumin and transferrin) and somatic body proteins (skeletal, smooth muscle, and tissue proteins).

  – These proteins and their amino acids are converted to glucose for energy (gluconeogenesis).

  – When these essential body proteins break down, a negative nitrogen balance results (more protein is used by the body than is taken in); starvation and disease-related stress contribute to this catabolic (destructive) state.

# Protein-energy malnutrition

## Key facts

- Protein-energy malnutrition (PEM) is essentially a deficiency of protein and calories (energy); it's also called *protein-calorie malnutrition*.
- PEM may be classified according to three forms: iatrogenic, kwashiorkor, and marasmus.

## What causes it

- Cancer
- GI disorders
- Chronic heart failure
- Alcoholism
- Conditions causing high metabolic needs such as burns

## What to consider

Protein-energy malnutrition can cause:

- reduced enzyme and plasma protein production
- increased susceptibility to infection
- physical and mental growth deficiencies in children
- severe diarrhea and malabsorption
- many secondary nutritional deficiencies
- delayed wound healing
- mental fatigue.

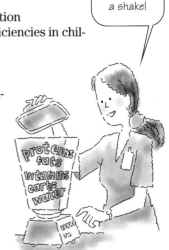

Now that's what I call a shake!

## Performing a nutritional assessment

## Obtaining a dietary history

What to do

- Look for signs of decreased food intake, increased metabolic requirements, or a combination of the two.
- Check the patient's dietary recall, using either a 24-hour food recall or diet diary.
- Obtain a thorough patient and family history, including major illnesses, hospitalizations, or known genetic conditions.
- Obtain the patient's weight history; note large weight gains or losses and when they occurred.
- Note factors that affect food intake and changes in appetite such as emotional events.
- Ask the patient about allergies and intolerances to foods or medications.
- Assess for psychosocial or environmental factors that may affect eating, such as limited or low income, use of tobacco or illicit drugs, limited community resources, living alone, or lack of transportation.

# Performing a physical assessment

## What to do

- Assess the patient's chief complaint, present illness, and over-all condition, including an inspection of his skin, mouth, and teeth.
- Obtain the patient's current weight, comparing it with his weight history.
- Review the patient's past medical history, noting previous major illnesses, injuries, hospitalizations, and surgeries.
- Review the patient's family history, paying particular attention to familial, genetic, or environmental illnesses.

## What to look for

In a patient with suspected nutrition problems, look for:
- abdominal masses and tenderness and an enlarged liver
- abnormal pigmentation
- adventitious breath sounds
- darkening of the oral mucosa
- dental caries
- exophthalmos
- ill-fitting dentures
- muscle wasting
- neck swelling
- poor skin turgor
- signs of infection or irritation on the roof of the mouth.

# Anthropometry

## Key facts

- Objective, noninvasive method for measuring overall body size, composition, and specific body parts
- Compares the patient's measurements with established standards

---

### Help desk

## Taking anthropometric measurements

**Arm midpoint**
Locate the midpoint on the patient's upper arm by placing a nonstretching tape measure between the acromion process of the scapula and the olecranon process of the ulna; mark the midpoint with a marking pen.

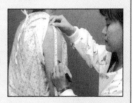

**Triceps skin-fold thickness**
Determine the triceps skin-fold thickness by grasping the patient's skin between the thumb and forefinger approximately 1 cm above the midpoint. Place the calipers at the midpoint and squeeze them for about 3 seconds. Record the measurement registered on the handle gauge to the nearest 0.5 mm. Take two more readings, then average all three to compensate for possible error.

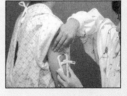

(continued)

**Taking anthropometric measurements** *(continued)*

**Midarm and midarm muscle circumferences**
At the marked midpoint, measure the midarm circumference. Calculate midarm muscle circumference by multiplying the triceps skin-fold thickness (in centimeters) by 3.143 and subtracting the result from the midarm circumference.

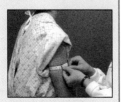

Compare the patient's measurements with the standard. A measurement less than 90% of the standard indicates calorie deprivation; a measurement more than 90% of the standard indicates adequate or more-than-adequate energy reserves.

| Measurement | Standard | 90% |
|---|---|---|
| Midarm circumference | Men: 29.3 cm <br> Women: 26.5 cm | Men: 26.4 cm <br> Women: 23.9 cm |
| Triceps skin-fold thickness | Men: 12.5 mm <br> Women: 16.5 mm | Men: 11.3 mm <br> Women: 14.9 mm |
| Midarm muscle circumference | Men: 25.3 cm <br> Women 23.2 cm | Men: 22.8 cm <br> Women: 20.9 cm |

- Commonly used anthropometric measurements:
  - height
  - weight
  - ideal body weight
  - body frame size
  - triceps skinfold thickness
  - midarm circumference
  - midarm muscle circumference
- Findings of less than 90% of standard measurement indicate possible need for nutritional support

# Diagnostic studies

## Key facts

- Used to evaluate visceral protein status, lean body mass, vitamin and mineral balance, and nutritional support effectiveness

### Detecting nutritional deficiencies

| Test and purpose | Normal findings | Implications |
|---|---|---|
| **Creatinine height index**<br>• Uses a 24-hour urine sample to determine adequacy of muscle mass | • Determined from a reference table of values based on a patient's height or weight | • Less than 80% of reference value: moderate depletion of muscle mass (protein reserves)<br>• Less than 60% of reference value: severe depletion, with increased risk of compromised immune function |
| **Hematocrit**<br>• Diagnoses anemia and dehydration | • Male: 42% to 50%<br>• Female: 40% to 48%<br>• Child: 29% to 41% | • Increased: severe dehydration, polycythemia<br>• Decreased: iron deficiency anemia, excessive blood loss |
| **Hemoglobin**<br>• Assesses blood's oxygen-carrying capacity to aid diagnosis of anemia, protein deficiency, and hydration status | • Adult male: 13 to 18 g/dl<br>• Adult female: 12 to 16 g/dl<br>• Older adult: 10 to 17 g/dl<br>• Child: 9 to 15.5 g/dl | • Increased: dehydration, polycythemia<br>• Decreased: protein deficiency, iron deficiency anemia, excessive blood loss, overhydration |

(continued)

## Detecting nutritional deficiencies (continued)

| Test and purpose | Normal findings | Implications |
|---|---|---|
| **Serum albumin** • Helps assess visceral protein stores | • Adult: 3.5 to 5 g/dl • Child: 3.5 to 5 g/dl | • Decreased values: malnutrition, overhydration, liver or kidney disease, heart failure, excessive blood loss such as from severe burns |
| **Serum transferrin** • Similar to serum total iron binding capacity (TIBC) • Helps assess visceral protein stores • Has a shorter half-life than serum albumin and, thus, more accurately reflects current status | • Adult: 200 to 400 mcg/dl • Child: 350 to 450 mcg/dl | • Increased TIBC: iron deficiency, as in pregnancy or iron deficiency anemia • Decreased TIBC: iron excess, as in chronic inflammatory states • Below 200 mcg/dl: visceral protein depletion • Below 100 mcg/dl: severe visceral protein depletion |
| **Serum triglycerides** • Screens for hyperlipidemia | • 40 to 200 mg/dl | • Increased values combined with increased cholesterol levels: increased risk of atherosclerotic disease • Decreased values: PEM, steatorrhea |

## Detecting nutritional deficiencies (continued)

| Test and purpose | Normal findings | Implications |
|---|---|---|
| **Total lymphocyte count**<br>• Diagnoses PEM | • 1,500 to 3,000/µl | • Increased values: infection or inflammation, leukemia, tissue necrosis<br>• Decreased values: moderate to severe malnutrition if no other cause, such as influenza or measles, identified |
| **Total protein screen**<br>• Detects hyperproteinemia or hypoproteinemia | • 6 to 8 g/dl | • Increased values: dehydration<br>• Decreased values: malnutrition, protein loss |
| **Transthyretin**<br>• Known as *prealbumin*<br>• Offers information regarding visceral protein stores<br>• Should be used in conjunction with albumin level<br>• Sensitive to nutritional depletion | • 16 to 40 mg/dl | • Increased values: renal insufficiency, patient on dialysis<br>• Decreased values: PEM, acute catabolic states, postsurgery, hyperthyroidism |
| **Urine ketone bodies**<br>• Screens for ketonuria and detects carbohydrate deprivation | • Negative for ketones in urine | • Ketoacidosis: starvation |

## Types of parenteral nutrition solutions

## Total parenteral nutrition (TPN)

### Key facts

- Common solutions include:
  - dextrose, 20% to 70% (1 L dextrose 25% = 850 nonprotein calories)
  - crystalline amino acids, 2.5% to 15%
  - electrolytes, vitamins, micronutrients, insulin, and heparin
  - lipid emulsion, 10% or 20%
  - water.

### Why it's used

- Provides long-term therapy (3 weeks or longer) to:
  - supply large quantities of nutrients and calories (2,000 to 2,500 calories/day or more)
  - restore nitrogen balance and replace essential vitamins, electrolytes, minerals, and trace elements
  - promote tissue synthesis, wound healing, and normal metabolic function
  - allow bowel rest and healing, reduce activity in the pancreas and small intestine
  - improve tolerance to surgery if severely malnourished.

### What to consider

- Considered nutritionally complete
- Requires minor surgical procedure for central venous catheter insertion
- May result in glucose intolerance or electrolyte imbalances from hypertonic solution
- May not be effective in severely stressed patients (such as those with sepsis or burns)
- May interfere with immune mechanisms

# Peripheral parenteral nutrition (PPN)

## Key facts

- Common solutions include:
  - dextrose, 5% to 10%
  - crystalline amino acids, 2.75% to 4.25%
  - electrolytes, minerals, micronutrients, and vitamins
  - lipid emulsion, 10% or 20%.

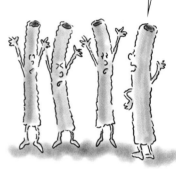

OK, guys, we really need to get into shape if we're gonna pull this one off...now stretch those tunicae!

## Why it's used

- Provides short-term therapy (3 weeks or less) to maintain nutritional state in patients who:
  - can tolerate a relatively high fluid volume
  - usually resume bowel function and oral feedings in a few days
  - aren't candidates for central venous catheters.
- Provides approximately 1,300 to 1,800 calories/day.

## What to consider

- Considered nutritionally complete for short-term therapy
- Shouldn't be used in nutritionally depleted patients
- Can't be used in volume-restricted patients because it requires high volumes of solution
- Doesn't cause weight gain
- Avoids insertion and maintenance of a central venous catheter
- Delivers less hypertonic solutions
- May cause phlebitis
- Lower risk of metabolic complications

## Components of parenteral nutrition solutions

### Amino acids

- Supplying enough protein to:
  - replace essential amino acids
  - maintain protein stores
  - prevent protein loss from muscle tissues.

### Dextrose

- Provides most of the calories needed to help maintain nitrogen balance
- Number of nonprotein calories needed to maintain nitrogen balance depends on the severity of the patient's illness

### Electrolytes and minerals

- Added to solution based on patient's serum chemistry profile and metabolic needs

### Fats

- Supplied as lipid emulsions to:
  - correct fatty acid deficiencies
  - provide up to 50% of a patient's caloric intake
- Available in several concentrations

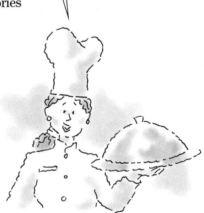

Today's special is a parenteral delight — some lovely amino acids with a touch of dextrose and a sprinkle of electrolytes and minerals, with just a hint of vitamins and water.

## Micronutrients
- Also called *trace elements*
- Promote normal metabolism
- Most commercial solutions contain zinc, copper, chromium, selenium, and manganese

## Vitamins
- Ensure normal body functions and optimal nutrient use for the patient
- Commercially available mixture of fat- and water-soluble vitamins, biotin, and folic acid may be added to parenteral nutrition solution

## Water
- Added to a parenteral nutrition solution based on fluid requirements and electrolyte balance

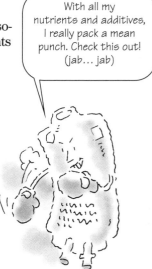

With all my nutrients and additives, I really pack a mean punch. Check this out! (jab... jab)

## Common additives
Depending on the patient's condition, additives may be ordered to treat a patient's specific metabolic deficiencies:
- acetate — prevents metabolic acidosis
- amino acids — provide protein necessary for tissue repair
- calcium — promotes development of bones and teeth; aids in blood clotting
- chloride — regulates acid-base equilibrium; maintains osmotic pressure
- dextrose 50% in water — provides calories for metabolism

- folic acid—essential for deoxyribonucleic acid formation; promotes growth and development
- magnesium—aids carbohydrate and protein absorption
- micronutrients (zinc, manganese, cobalt)—help in wound healing and red blood cell synthesis
- phosphate—minimizes potential for developing peripheral paresthesia (numbness and tingling of the extremities)
- potassium—essential for cellular activity and tissue synthesis
- sodium—helps regulate water distribution and maintain normal fluid balance
- vitamin B complex—aids final absorption of carbohydrates and protein
- vitamin C—helps in wound healing
- vitamin D—essential for bone metabolism and maintenance of serum calcium levels
- vitamin K—helps prevent bleeding disorders.

## Total nutrient admixture
- A milky white solution that delivers 1 day's worth of nutrients in a single 3-L bag
- Also called *3:1 solution*
- Combines lipids with other parenteral solution components

### Benefits to using total nutrient admixture
- Less need to handle the bag (less risk of contamination)
- Less time required to set up and prepare for administration
- Less need for infusion sets and electronic infusion devices
- Lower facility costs
- Increased patient mobility
- Easier adjustment to home care

## Drawbacks to using total nutrient admixture

- Use of certain infusion devices precluded because of their inability to accurately deliver large volumes of solution
- 1.2-micron filter required (rather than a 0.22-micron filter) to allow lipid molecules through
- Limited amount of calcium and phosphorus added because of the difficulty in detecting precipitate in the milky white solution

## Lipid emulsions

- Lipid emulsions are administered only with TPN.
- In oral diets, lipids or fats are the major source of calories (usually 40% of total caloric intake).
- In TPN solutions, lipids provide 9 kcal/g.
- I.V. lipid emulsions are oxidized for energy as needed.
- As a nearly isotonic emulsion, concentrations of 10% or 20% can be safely infused through peripheral or central veins.
- Lipid emulsions prevent and treat essential fatty acid deficiency and provide a major source of energy.

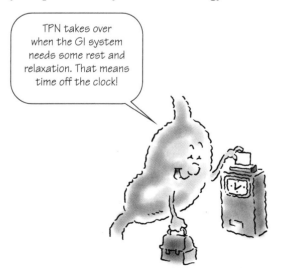

## Managing parenteral nutrition

## Maintaining a TPN infusion

### Key facts

- Intake increased by doctor to the goal rate on the second day if patient tolerates solution well on the first day

### What to do

- Check the doctor's order against the TPN container's label.
- Label the container with the expiration date, time the solution was hung, glucose concentration, and total volume of solution. (If the bag or bottle is damaged and you don't have an immediate replacement, you can approximate the glucose concentration until a new container is ready by adding 50% glucose to dextrose 10% in water.)
- Maintain flow rates as prescribed, even if the flow falls behind schedule.
- Don't allow TPN solutions to infuse for more than 24 hours.
- Change the tubing and filter every 24 hours, using strict aseptic technique; make sure that all tubing junctions are secure.
- Perform I.V. site care and dressing changes according to your facility's policy and protocol—usually every 48 hours, more often if the dressing becomes wet, soiled, or nonocclusive.
- Check the infusion pump's volume meter and time tape every 30 minutes (or more often, if necessary) to monitor for irregular flow rate; never use gravity to administer TPN.

Oops! Keep in mind that gravity and TPN don't mix.

- Record vital signs when you initiate therapy and every 4 to 8 hours thereafter (or more often, if necessary).
- Be alert for increased body temperature — one of the earliest signs of catheter-related sepsis.
- Accurately record the patient's daily fluid intake and output, specifying the volume and type of each fluid.
- Assess the patient's physical status daily.
- Suspect fluid imbalance if the patient gains more than 1 lb (0.45 kg) per day.
- Monitor the results of routine laboratory tests, such as serum electrolyte, blood urea nitrogen, and glucose levels, and report abnormal findings to the doctor so appropriate changes in the TPN solution can be made.
- Check serum triglyceride levels, which should be in the normal range during continuous TPN infusion.
- Make sure that alanine aminotransferase, aspartate aminotransferase, alkaline phosphatase, cholesterol, triglyceride, plasma-free fatty acid, and coagulation tests are performed weekly, or as ordered.
- Monitor the patient for signs and symptoms of nutritional aberrations, such as fluid and electrolyte imbalances and glucose metabolism disturbances.
- Provide emotional support.
- Provide frequent mouth care.

Remember to check all laboratory studies carefully...you don't want to gamble that everything's normal when some adjustments might need to be made.

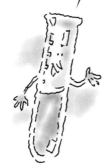

# Maintaining a PPN infusion

## Key facts

- Involves same steps as for any patient receiving peripheral I.V. infusion

## What to do

- Maintain the infusion rate and care for tubing, dressing, site, and I.V. devices.
- Monitor the patient for an allergic reaction to the lipid emulsion.
- Monitor the patient for signs and symptoms of sepsis, including:
  - glucose in the urine (glycosuria)
  - chills
  - malaise
  - increased white blood cells (leukocytosis)
  - altered level of consciousness
  - elevated glucose levels (measured by fingerstick or serum chemistry)
  - elevated temperature.
- Monitor the patient for early signs and symptoms of adverse reactions to lipid emulsion therapy, including:
  - fever
  - difficulty breathing
  - cyanosis
  - nausea
  - vomiting
  - headache
  - flushing
  - sweating
  - lethargy
  - dizziness
  - chest and back pain
  - slight pressure over the eyes
  - irritation at the infusion site.

## What to consider

- Because the synthesis of lipase (a fat-splitting enzyme) increases insulin requirements, the insulin dosage of a patient with diabetes may need to be increased as ordered. (Insulin is one of the additives that may need to be adjusted in the patient's peripheral parenteral nutrition solution.)
- For a patient with hypothyroidism, you may need to administer thyroid-stimulating hormone (affects lipase activity and may prevent triglycerides from accumulating in the vascular system).
- Patients receiving lipid emulsions commonly report a feeling of fullness or bloating; occasionally, they experience an unpleasant metallic or greasy taste.

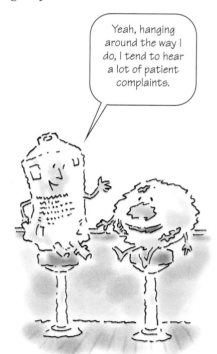

Yeah, hanging around the way I do, I tend to hear a lot of patient complaints.

# Managing problems in parenteral therapy

- Includes:
  - troubleshooting problems with I.V. infusion setups
  - problems with weaning patient from TPN or PPN therapy.

## Discontinuing parenteral therapy

Key facts

- Wean the patient off TPN over 24 hours to prevent rebound hypoglycemia; don't abruptly discontinue TPN.
- Before weaning, provide another form of nutritional therapy (such as enteral feedings).
- Avoid weaning a patient before discontinuing PPN therapy as the dextrose concentration is lower than in TPN.

*Smooth sailing*

### Troubleshooting problems with parenteral infusion setups

| Problem and signs and symptoms | What to do |
| --- | --- |
| **Clotted catheter** <br> • Interrupted infusion flow rate <br> • Greater pressure needed to maintain the infusion at the desired infusion rate | • Reposition the catheter and attempt to aspirate the clot; if unsuccessful, instill alteplase to clear the catheter lumen as ordered. |

**Troubleshooting problems with parenteral infusion setups**
*(continued)*

| Problem and signs and symptoms | What to do |
|---|---|
| *Cracked or broken tubing*<br>• Dry I.V. insertion site<br>• Infusate leaking from the insertion site or cracked area | • Apply a padded hemostat above the break to prevent air from entering the line. |
| *Dislodged catheter*<br>• Bleeding from the insertion site and air embolism (most significant)<br>• Patient reports a wet gown or feeling cold<br>• Wet dressing<br>• Catheter located peripherally — area around the insertion site may be red or swollen due to subcutaneous extravasation of the solution<br>• Centrally inserted catheter — possible swelling or redness around the insertion site | • Place a sterile gauze pad on the insertion site, and apply pressure. |
| *Overly rapid infusion*<br>• Headache<br>• Heart failure due to fluid overload<br>• Lethargy<br>• Nausea | • Check the infusion rate.<br>• Check the infusion pump. |

# Managing patients with special needs

## Pediatric patients

### Key facts

- Parenteral feeding therapy for children maintains a child's nutritional status and fuels a child's growth.
- Children have a greater need for nutrients than adults, including:
  - carbohydrates
  - electrolytes
  - fat
  - fluids
  - micronutrients
  - protein
  - vitamins.
- Administering PPN with lipid emulsions in a premature or low-birth-weight neonate may lead to lipid accumulation in the lungs. Thrombocytopenia (platelet deficiency) has also been reported in neonates receiving 20% lipid emulsions.

### What to do

- Keep in mind these factors when planning to meet children's nutritional needs:
  - age
  - weight
  - activity level
  - body proportion
  - development
  - caloric needs.

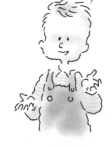

Kids aren't small adults. We're special people with special needs — including our need for nutrients.

# Elderly patients

## Key facts

- Elderly patients are at risk for fluid overload when receiving TPN or PPN.
- An elderly patient may have underlying clinical problems that affect the outcome of treatment. For example, he may be taking medications that can interact with the components in the parenteral nutrition solution.

## What to do

- Monitor flow rates carefully to prevent complications associated with overinfusion.

### *Help desk*

### Fluid overload

Pediatric and elderly patients are particularly susceptible to fluid overload and heart failure. With these patients, be particularly careful to administer the correct volume of parenteral nutrition solution at the correct infusion rate.

## Managing complications

## Air embolism

### Key facts

- Mechanical complication
- Potentially fatal
- Can occur during I.V. tubing changes if the tubing is inadvertently disconnected
- Can also result from undetected hairline cracks in the tubing

### What to look for

- Apprehension
- Cardiac arrest
- Chest pain
- Churning heart murmur (classic sign)
- Cyanosis
- Loss of consciousness
- Hypotension
- Seizures
- Tachycardia

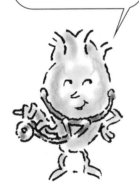

Yikes! Do you hear that churning murmur? It's a classic sign of air embolism from parenteral therapy!

### What to do

- Clamp the catheter.
- Place the patient on his left side in Trendelenburg's position.
- Give oxygen as ordered.
- If cardiac arrest occurs, use cardiopulmonary resuscitation.

### How to prevent it

- Be sure to secure all tubing connections.
- Maintain the integrity of the occlusive dressing.

# Hyperglycemia

## Key facts

- Metabolic complication
- May develop if the formula's glucose concentration is excessive, the infusion rate is too rapid, or glucose tolerance is compromised by diabetes, stress, or sepsis

## What to look for

- Anxiety
- Coma
- Confusion
- Dehydration
- Delirium
- Elevated blood and urine glucose levels
- Fatigue
- Polyuria
- Restlessness
- Weakness

## What to do

- Start insulin therapy or adjust the TPN flow rate as ordered.

## How to prevent it

- Monitor serum glucose levels every 6 hours initially.
- Maintain serum glucose levels less than 200 mg/dl.
- Initiate the infusion slowly, using an infusion pump.

# Hyperkalemia

### Key facts

- Metabolic complication
- Develops because of too much potassium in the TPN formula, renal disease, or hyponatremia

### What to look for

- Decreased heart rate
- Irregular pulse
- Skeletal muscle weakness
- Tall T waves

### What to do

- Decrease potassium supplementation.

### How to prevent it

- Monitor serum electrolyte levels daily at the initiation of therapy.

Too much K in the TPN can cause a P.R.O.B.L.E.M. — hyperkalemia, to be specific.

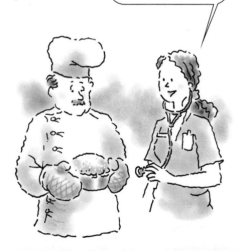

# Hypoglycemia

## Key facts

- Metabolic complication
- May develop if parenteral nutrition is interrupted suddenly or if patient receives excessive insulin

## What to look for

- Confusion
- Irritability
- Shaking
- Sweating

## What to do

- Infuse dextrose as ordered.

## How to prevent it

- Monitor serum glucose levels every 6 hours initially.
- When discontinuing TPN, decrease the infusion slowly.

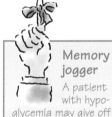

**Memory jogger**

A patient with hypoglycemia may give off signs that he needs something sweet — such as a chocolate "Ciss" (remember **"C,"** not a **"K"**), or at least a little glucose in his infusion:

Confusion

Irritability

Shaking

Sweating.

# Hypokalemia

## Key facts

- Metabolic complication
- Develops because of too little potassium in the solution, excessive loss of potassium brought on by GI tract disturbances or diuretic use, or large doses of insulin

## What to look for

- Cardiac arrhythmias
- Muscle weakness
- Paralysis
- Paresthesia

## What to do

- Increase potassium supplementation.

## How to prevent it

- Monitor severely malnourished patients for refeeding syndrome.
- Initiate feeding slowly and monitor electrolyte levels.

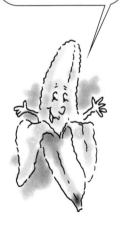

Whenever people talk about too little potassium, they usually point to me — I'm the scapegoat. But as you can see, hypokalemia can result from nondietary factors, too.

# Hypomagnesemia

## Key facts
- Metabolic complication
- Results from insufficient magnesium in the solution

## What to look for
- Cardiac arrhythmias
- Hyperreflexia
- Mental changes
- Paresthesia in the fingers
- Tetany
- Tingling around the mouth

## What to do
- Increase magnesium supplementation.

## How to prevent it
- Monitor severely malnourished patients for refeeding syndrome.
- Initiate feeding slowly and monitor electrolyte levels.

# Metabolic acidosis

## Key facts
- Metabolic complication
- Can occur if the patient develops an increased serum chloride level and a decreased serum bicarbonate level

## What to look for
- Confusion
- Dull headache
- Hypotension
- Kussmaul's respirations
- Lethargy
- Warm, dry skin

## What to do
- Use acetate or lactate salts of sodium or hydrogen to buffer acidosis.

## How to prevent it
- Monitor serum chloride and bicarbonate levels.
- Closely monitor electrolyte levels while the condition is corrected.

# Phlebitis

## Key facts
- Mechanical complication
- Also known as *inflammation of a vein*

## What to look for
- Pain
- Redness
- Tenderness
- Warmth at the insertion site and along the vein path

## What to do
- Apply moderate heat to the insertion site.
- Elevate the insertion site, if possible.

## How to prevent it
- Assess the insertion site frequently for redness and swelling.
- Monitor the patient's pain level.

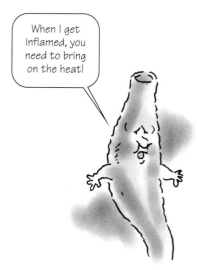

When I get inflamed, you need to bring on the heat!

# Sepsis

## Key facts
- The most serious catheter-related complication
- Can be fatal

## What to look for
- Chills
- Red, indurated area around the catheter site
- Unexplained fever
- Unexplained hyperglycemia (usually an early warning sign)

## What to do
- Remove the catheter and culture the tip.
- Give antibiotics as ordered.

## How to prevent it
- Maintain meticulous and consistent aseptic technique during catheter insertion, site dressing changes, and tubing changes.

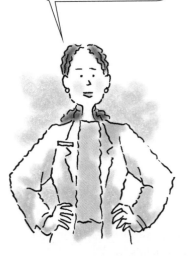

Sepsis is no laughing matter. Unexplained fever or hyperglycemia can be warning signs of the most serious catheter-related complication.

# Venous thrombosis

## Key facts
- Mechanical complication
- Can occur secondary to vein wall trauma during insertion
- Can also result from catheter movement against the vein wall after insertion

## What to look for
- Fever
- Malaise
- Pain at the insertion site and along the vein
- Redness or swelling at the catheter insertion site
- Swelling of the arm, neck, or face
- Tachycardia

## What to do
- Remove the catheter promptly.
- Administer heparin, if ordered.
- Perform venous flow studies, if appropriate.

## How to prevent it
- Use a stabilization board.
- Properly secure the catheter.
- Perform careful insertion, minimizing catheter manipulation.

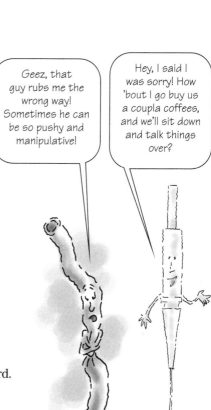

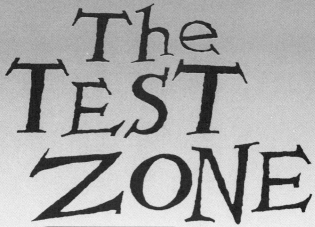

# The TEST ZONE

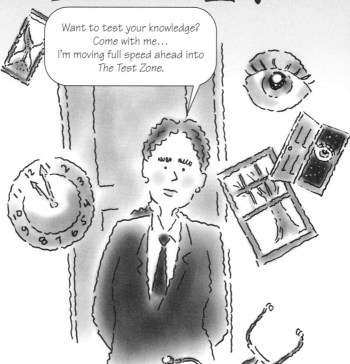

Want to test your knowledge?
Come with me…
I'm moving full speed ahead into
*The Test Zone*.

## Chapter 1: Fundamentals of I.V. therapy

**1.** Your patient shows signs and symptoms of diminished urine output, poor skin turgor, thirst, and dry, cracked lips. These symptoms would most likely indicate:
  A. fluid excess.
  B. fluid deficit.
  C. hyperkalemia.
  D. hypokalemia.

**2.** An I.V. solution with an osmolarity higher than that of serum is called:
  A. isotonic.
  B. hypotonic.
  C. hypertonic.
  D. ionic.

**3.** The best type of I.V. delivery method for patients requiring a low volume of fluid is:
  A. intermittent infusion using a volume-control set.
  B. intermittent infusion using a saline lock.
  C. direct injection through an existing infusion line.
  D. direct injection into a vein.

**4.** An example of an isotonic I.V. solution is:
  A. dextrose 5% in half-normal saline.
  B. 25% albumin.
  C. dextrose 2.5% in water.
  D. 5% albumin.

## Chapter 2: Peripheral I.V. therapy

**5.** In pediatric patients, scalp veins are extremely fragile. They should be used only with patients younger than age:

   A. 6 months.

   B. 12 months.

   C. 18 months.

   D. 2 years.

**6.** What's a disadvantage to using the median antebrachial vein for a peripheral venipuncture site?

   A. It's difficult to splint the elbow area with an arm board.

   B. It decreases wrist movement.

   C. It has a high risk of infiltration.

   D. It's difficult for the patient to eat with the device in place.

**7.** If you detect signs of infection when you change your patient's peripheral I.V. dressing, the most important nursing intervention would be to:

   A. notify the doctor.

   B. redress the I.V. site.

   C. monitor the I.V. site frequently.

   D. remove the catheter or needle.

**8.** Which measure should you take to prevent hematoma at the venipuncture site?

   A. Choose a vein that accommodates the size of venous access device.

   B. Use a pump or controller for I.V. fluids.

   C. Purge the tubing of air completely before insertion.

   D. Tape the device securely to prevent movement.

## Chapter 3: Central venous therapy

**9.** The purpose of the Dacron cuff on CV catheters is to:
  A. allow sampling of blood.
  B. allow infusion of multiple solutions.
  C. eliminate the need for heparin flushes.
  D. prevent bacterial migration.

**10.** Your patient has a subclavian CV catheter. You should monitor him most closely for:
  A. kinked catheter.
  B. pneumothorax.
  C. thrombus.
  D. wound dressing placement.

**11.** Which situation is an appropriate indication for a short-term, single-lumen catheter?
  A. To use in home therapy
  B. To help a patient with heparin allergy
  C. To achieve emergency access
  D. To help a patient with small central vessels

**12.** After removing a CV catheter from a subclavian vein, a dry dressing should be maintained over the site for:
  A. 12 hours.
  B. 24 hours.
  C. 48 hours.
  D. 72 hours.

## Chapter 4: I.V. medications

**13.** Your patient weighs 165 lb. In order to calculate the dosage of his I.V. medication you must convert his weight to kilograms (kg). His weight in kg would be:
  A. 0.75 kg.
  B. 7.5 kg.
  C. 75 kg.
  D. 750 kg.

**14.** A systemic reaction that may occur when I.V. infusions are administered too quickly is known as:
  A. systemic infection.
  B. venous spasm.
  C. anaphylactic shock.
  D. speed shock.

**15.** What's the main indication for intermittent infusion using the piggyback method?
  A. To administer drugs given over short periods at varying intervals
  B. To administer a drug that's incompatible with an I.V. solution
  C. To maintain continuous serum levels
  D. For immediate drug effect in emergencies

**16.** What's the most common method of giving I.V. drugs to pediatric patients?
  A. Continuous infusion through a primary line
  B. Intermittent infusion using a volume-control set
  C. Intermittent infusion using a saline lock
  D. Intermittent infusion using the piggyback method

## Chapter 5: Transfusions

**17.** What's the maximum amount of time a unit of packed RBCs may infuse?

    A. 2 hours

    B. 3 hours

    C. 4 hours

    D. 5 hours

**18.** Signs and symptoms of a hemolytic reaction include blood oozing at the infusion site, chills, and:

    A. oliguria.

    B. urticaria.

    C. abdominal pain.

    D. hypertension.

**19.** To help prevent hypocalcemia in the patient receiving a blood transfusion, the nurse should:

    A. infuse the blood rapidly.

    B. infuse the blood slowly.

    C. premedicate the patient with an antipyretic.

    D. monitor the electrocardiogram.

**20.** A patient is typed and crossed matched for packed RBCs and is found to be type A. What blood type should she receive?

    A. O only

    B. AB, A, B, or O

    C. B or O

    D. A or O

## Chapter 6: Chemotherapy infusions

**21.** If your patient develops a hypersensitivity reaction to chemotherapy, the emergency drugs usually administered first are:
    A. antipyretics.
    B. bronchodilators.
    C. antihistamines.
    D. corticosteroids.

**22.** Cycle-specific chemotherapy drugs are:
    A. able to act on both reproducing and resting cells.
    B. divided into five categories.
    C. responsible for a fixed percentage of normal and malignant cells dying during a single administration.
    D. designed to disrupt a specific biochemical process.

**23.** What's the best way to assess peripheral I.V. placement for a patient receiving chemotherapy infusions?
    A. Check for blood return.
    B. Observe the site for swelling during chemotherapy infusion.
    C. Observe the site for swelling after normal saline solution flush.
    D. Ask the patient if the I.V. site is tender.

**24.** What's the primary function of interleukins, a type of immunomodulatory cytokines?
    A. Reduce the incidence of infection in patients receiving chemotherapeutic drugs.
    B. Induce erythroid maturation.
    C. Play a role in inflammatory response to tumors.
    D. Deliver messages to leukocytes.

## Chapter 7: Parenteral nutrition

**25.** What would be the most appropriate nursing intervention if you suspect cracked or broken tubing while administering parenteral therapy to a patient?
- A. Place a sterile gauze over the insertion site.
- B. Slow the infusion rate.
- C. Apply a padded hemostat above the break.
- D. Notify the doctor.

**26.** Your patient is receiving TPN and is complaining of tingling around his mouth and paresthesia in his fingers. These symptoms are most likely caused by:
- A. hyperkalemia.
- B. metabolic acidosis.
- C. hypoglycemia.
- D. hypomagnesemia.

**27.** What percentage of lipid emulsions can be safely infused through peripheral veins?
- A. 20%
- B. 25%
- C. 30%
- D. 40%

**28.** Which parenteral nutrition solution is most appropriate for short-term therapy?
- A. PPN
- B. TPN
- C. Total nutrient admixture
- D. Lipid emulsion

# Answers

## Chapter 1: Fundamentals of I.V. therapy

**1.** B. In addition to those listed, indications of fluid deficit include decreased central venous pressure, mental status changes, and weakness.

**2.** C. Hypertonic solutions have higher osmolarity than serum and draw fluid into intravascular compartment from the cells and interstitial compartments. Examples of these solutions are dextrose 5% in water and dextrose 5% in lactated Ringers.

**3.** A. Intermittent infusions using a volume-control set are best used for low volume fluid infusions because they require only one large volume container and prevent fluid overload from runaway infusion.

**4.** D. Isotonic solutions osmolarity is about equal to that of serum; 5% albumin is 308 mOsm/L.

## Chapter 2: Peripheral I.V. therapy

**5.** A. Because scalp veins are extremely fragile, they should be used only in infants younger than age 6 months. An older child is more likely to move his head and dislodge the venipuncture device.

**6.** C. The median antebrachial vein runs along the ulnar side of the forearm and has a high risk of infiltration.

**7.** D. If you detect signs or phlebitis, apply pressure to the area with a sterile gauze pad and remove the catheter or needle.

**8.** A. Choosing the appropriate vein for the size of the venous access device will decrease the chance of leakage of blood into tissue leading to hematoma.

## Chapter 3: Central venous therapy

**9.** D. The Dacron cuff, found on Groshong, Hickman, and Broviac catheters, prevents excess motion and organism migration.

**10.** B. Because of close proximity to major thoracic organs, a patient with a CV catheter in the subclavian site must be monitored for dyspnea, shortness of breath, and sudden chest pain.

**11.** C. Because it can be inserted at the bedside and its stiffness aids in CV pressure monitoring, the short-term, single-lumen catheter is indicated as an emergency CV access.

**12.** D. Some vessels, such as the subclavian vein, aren't easily compressed. By 72 hours the site should be sealed and the risk of air embolism should be past.

## Chapter 4: I.V. medications

**13.** C. Knowing that 2.2 lb = 1 kg, divide 165 by 2.2 to convert pounds to kilograms.

**14.** D. This complication can be prevented by administering I.V. fluids at the prescribed rate, never speeding up a medication infusion, and using an I.V. pump for precise delivery of a medication.

**15.** A. Intermittent infusion using the piggyback method is indicated for drugs given over short periods at varying intervals, such as antibiotics and gastric-secretion inhibitors.

**16.** B. Intermittent infusion using a volume-control set is the most common method for children because children are more prone to fluid overload; volume control sets help prevent a runaway infusion.

## Chapter 5: Transfusions

**17.** C. Transfusions usually shouldn't take longer than 4 hours because the risk of contamination and sepsis increases after that time. Discard or return to the blood bank any blood not given within this time, as your facility's policy directs.

**18.** A. Hemolytic reactions occur as a result of incompatible blood and may progress to shock and renal failure.

**19.** B. Hypocalcemia can be caused by citrate toxicity if the blood is infused too rapidly because citrate binds with calcium.

**20.** D. The patient who has type A blood can receive packed RBCs that are cross-matched either A or O.

## Chapter 6: Chemotherapy infusions

**21.** C. The specific treatment for a hypersensitivity reaction will depend on the severity of the reaction. Antihistamines are typically given first, followed by corticosteroids and bronchodilators.

**22.** D. Cycle-specific chemotherapy drugs are designed to disrupt a specific biochemical process, making them effective only during a specific phase of the cycle.

**23.** C. Blood return is an inconclusive test and shouldn't be used to determine if the I.V. catheter is placed correctly in the peripheral vein. Flush the vein with normal saline solution and observe for site swelling.

**24.** D. Interleukins' primarily function is to deliver messages to leukocytes.

## Chapter 7: Parenteral nutrition

**25.** C. Applying a padded hemostat above the break will help prevent air from entering the line.

**26.** D. Tingling around the mouth and paresthesia in the fingers are signs of hypomagnesemia, which can result from insufficient magnesium in the solution. Additional signs and symptoms include mental changes, hyperreflexia, tetany, and arrhythmias.

**27.** A. As a nearly isotonic emulsion, concentrations of 10% or 20% can be safely infused through peripheral or central veins.

**28.** A. PPN is used for short-term therapy (3 weeks or less) to maintain adequate nutrition in patients who can tolerate relatively high fluid volume and who usually resume bowel function and oral feedings in a few days.

## *Scoring*

☆☆☆ If you answered 25 to 28 questions correctly, great job! You're in a dimension all by yourself.

☆☆ If you answered 19 to 24 questions correctly, way to go! You're really in the zone.

☆ If you answered fewer than 19 questions correctly, review the chapters and try again! It won't be long until you see the light.

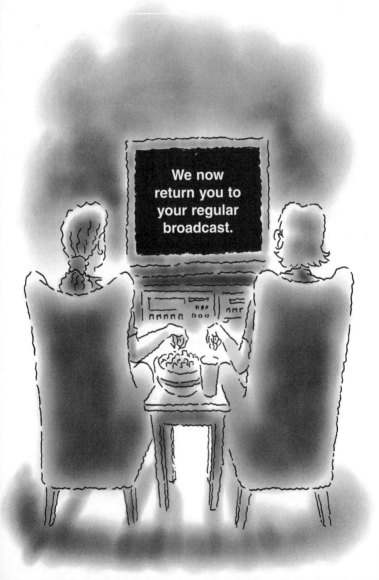

# Selected references

Alexander, M., and Corrigan, A.M., eds. *Core Curriculum for Infusion Nursing*, 3rd ed. Philadelphia: Lippincott Williams & Wilkins, 2003.

Evans-Smith, P. *Taylor's Clinical Nursing Skills: A Nursing Process Approach.* Philadelphia: Lippincott Williams & Wilkins, 2004.

Fernandez, R.S., et al. "Peripheral Venous Catheters: A Review of Current Practices," *Journal of Infusion Nursing* 26(6):388-92, November-December 2003.

Fiaccadori E., et al. "Enteral Nutrition in Patients With Acute Renal Failure," *Kidney International* 65(3):999-1008, March 2004.

Finlay, T. *Intravenous Therapy*, Malden, Mass.: Blackwell Publishing, 2004.

Gahart, B.L., and Nazareno, A.R. *2005 Intravenous Medications: A Handbook for Nurses and Allied Health Professionals*, 21st ed. Philadelphia: Mosby–Year Book, Inc., 2005.

Gorski, L.A. "Central Venous Access Device Occlusions: Part 1: Thrombotic Causes and Treatment," *Home Healthcare Nurse* 21(2):115-21, February 2003.

Gorski, L.A. "Central Venous Access Device Occlusions: Part 2: Nonthrombotic Causes and Treatment," *Home Healthcare Nurse* 21(3):168-71, March 2003.

Hadaway, L.C. "Infusing Without Infecting," *Nursing2003* 33(10):58-63, October 2003.

Infusion Nurses Society. *Infusion Therapy in Clinical Practice*, 2nd ed. Philadelphia: W.B. Saunders Co., 2001.

*I.V. Therapy Made Incredibly Easy*, 3rd ed. Philadelphia: Lippincott Williams & Wilkins, 2005.

Josephson, D.L. *Intravenous Infusion Therapy for Nurses: Principles & Practice*, 2nd ed. Albany, N.Y.: Delmar Learning, 2003.

*Just the Facts: I.V. Therapy.* Philadelphia: Lippincott Williams & Wilkins, 2004.

*Nursing2005 Drug Handbook*, 25th ed. Philadelphia: Lippincott Williams & Wilkins, 2005.

*Nursing Procedures*, 4th ed. Philadelphia: Lippincott Williams & Wilkins, 2004.

*Nursing Procedures and Protocols.* Philadelphia: Lippincott Williams & Wilkins, 2003.

Skeel, R.T. *Handbook of Cancer Chemotherapy*, 6th ed. Philadelphia: Lippincott Williams & Wilkins, 2003.

# Index

## A

Accessory cephalic vein, 29i, 33
Acute lymphocytic leukemia, 228t
Administration rates, calculating, 153
Administration set, changing, 53
Adriamycin, 228t
Air embolism, 60, 120-121, 284
Albumin, in nutritional deficiencies, 268t
Albumin, 5% and 25%, 200
Alkylating agents, 225t
Allergic reaction, 61-62, 208
Alopecia, chemotherapy and, 247
Amino acids, in parenteral nutrition solutions, 272
Ammonia level, elevated, multiple transfusions and, 215
Analgesia, patient-controlled, 169
Anaphylactic reactions, chemotherapy and, 251-253
Androgens, chemotherapeutic, 226t
Anemia, chemotherapy and, 248
Anesthetic, for venipuncture, 44, 45i
Antecubital veins, 29i, 34
Anthropometry, 265-266, 265-266i
Antiandrogens, chemotherapeutic, 226t
Antibiotics, chemotherapeutic, 225t
Antiestrogens, chemotherapeutic, 226t
Antimetabolites, chemotherapeutic, 225t
Asparaginase, 225t

## B

Bacterial contamination reaction, blood transfusion and, 209
Basilic vein, 29i, 35, 98, 99i
Bilateral superficial temporal vein, 57i
Biological response modifiers, 229
Biological Safety Cabinet, 234
Bladder cancer, 228t
Bleeding tendencies, multiple transfusions and, 214
Bleomycin, 225t, 228t
Blood, whole, 184-185
Blood bag, empty, 207
Blood sample, obtaining, 48
Blood transfusion, 194. *See also* Transfusions.
    complications of, 206-213

Blood transfusion *(continued)*
    monitoring, 196
    precautions for, 198
    pressure cuff in, 197
    stopped, 205
Blood type compatibility, 184, 185t
Bolus injection, administering, 134-135
Bottle, adding drug to, 154
Breast cancer, 228t
Broviac catheter, 81, 87-88, 87i
Buffered saline, 200

## C

Calcium, 3
Carboplatin, 225t
Catheter. *See also specific type.*
    central, 82
    inserting, 46
    kinked, 144t
    long-line, 79-80, 95-96, 95i
    over-the-needle, 37-38, 37i
    peripherally inserted central, 79-80
    scalp vein, 58
    severed, 70
    short-term multilumen, 85-86, 85i
    short-term single-lumen, 83-84, 83i
    tunneled, 81
Catheter dislodgment, 63
Catheter gauges, 41t
Catheter migration, 144t
Catheter tubing, changing, 110
Cell cycle, and chemotherapeutic drugs, 222, 223i, 224
Cellular products, 184-191
Central venous catheter, 79-82
    disconnected, 116
    drawing blood from, 111-113
    configurations for, 83-96
    removing, 114-115
Central venous therapy, 77-148
    applying dressing in, 105
    changing catheter tubing in, 110
    changing dressing in, 106-107, 106i
    drawing blood in, 111-112, 113, 119
    flushing catheter in, 108-109
    managing common problems in, 116-128

i refers to an illustration; t refers to a table.

Central venous therapy *(continued)*
   monitoring in, 103-104
   preparing for, 97-102, 99i
   removing catheter in, 114-115
   selecting insertion line in, 97
   veins used in, 98, 99i, 100-102
Cephalic vein, 29i, 36, 98, 99i
Cervical cancer, 228t
Chemotherapy, 233-239, 246-258
Chemotherapy protocols, 227, 228t
Chemotherapy spill, 239
Chemotherapeutic drugs, 222-224, 225-226t
   administering, 240-245
   safe handling of, 235-239
Chevron method, for securing I.V. site, 49, 49i
Chloride, 4
Chylothorax, 122-123
Circulatory overload, 64, 173, 210
Cisplatin, 225t, 228t
Clamp, closed, 144t
Clot formation, 144t
Colony-stimulating factors, 231
Compatibility, 151-152, 184, 185t
Contact time, and drug incompatibility, 151
Contamination, bacterial, blood transfusion
   and, 209
Continuous infusion, 20-21, 155-156
Creatinine height index, 267t
Cyclophosphamide, 225t, 228t
Cytarabine, 225t
Cytokines, immunomodulatory, 231-232
Cytoprotective agents, chemotherapeutic, 226t

**D**

Dacarbazine, 228t
Daunorubicin, 228t
Delivery methods, comparing, 15-21
Dexrazoxane, 226t
Dextrose, in parenteral nutrition solutions, 272
Diarrhea, chemotherapy and, 249
Digital veins, 28, 29i
Direct injection, 15, 16, 157, 158, 163-164, 165
Documentation, 24-26
Dosages, calculating, 153
Dorsal venous network, 29i, 31
Doxorubicin, 225t, 228t
Drawing blood, 111-113, 119, 139-141
Dressings, 51-52, 105, 106-107, 106i

Drug compatibility, 151-152
Drug concentration, and drug
   incompatibility, 151
Drug dosages, calculating, 153
Drug therapy. *See* Medication therapy.

**E**

Electrolytes, 2-10
Electrolytes and minerals, in parenteral
   nutrition solutions, 272
Enzymes, chemotherapeutic, 225t
Erythropoietin, 231
Estramustine, 226t
Estrogens, chemotherapeutic, 226t
Etoposide, 228t
Evacuated technique, 140-141
Evacuated tube, 111-112
Extravasation, 143, 174-175, 250

**F**

Factors II, VII, IX, and X complex, 202
Factor VIII, 201
Fats, in parenteral nutrition solutions, 272
Febrile reaction, blood transfusion and, 211
Fibrin sheath formation, vascular access
   port therapy and, 146
Flow rates, calculating, 22, 23i
Floxuridine, 225t
Fluid imbalances, 9-10
Fluid overload, parenteral nutrition and, 283
Fluorouracil, 225t
Flushing solutions, in central venous therapy,
   108-109
Flutamide, 226t
Folic acid analogs, chemotherapeutic, 226t
Fresh frozen plasma, 199

**G**

Gonadotropin, 226t
Granulocyte colony-stimulating factor, 231
Granulocyte-macrophage colony-stimulating
   factor, 231
Groshong catheter, 81, 89-90, 89i

**H**

Hair loss, chemotherapy and, 247
Hematocrit, in nutritional deficiencies, 267t
Hematoma, 65, 206
Hemoglobin, 219, 267t

i refers to an illustration; t refers to a table.

Hemolytic reaction, blood transfusion and, 212
Hemosiderosis, multiple transfusions and, 216
Hemothorax, central venous therapy and, 122-123
Heparinized saline solution, 108
Herceptin, 230t
Hickman catheter, 81, 91-92, 91i
Hickman-Broviac catheter, 93-94, 93i
H method, for securing I.V. site, 49i, 50
Hodgkin's disease, 228t
Hormone inhibitors, chemotherapeutic, 226t
Hormones, chemotherapeutic, 226t
Hydrothorax, central venous therapy and, 122-123
Hydroxyurea, 225t
Hypercalcemia, 3
Hyperchloremia, 4
Hyperglycemia, parenteral nutrition and, 285
Hyperkalemia, 7, 286
Hypermagnesemia, 5
Hypernatremia, 8
Hyperphosphatemia, 6
Hypersensitivity reactions, 176, 251-253, 252t
Hypertonic solutions, 11i, 13
Hypocalcemia, 3, 217
Hypochloremia, 4
Hypoglycemia, parenteral nutrition and, 287
Hypokalemia, 7, 288
Hypomagnesemia, 5, 289
Hyponatremia, 8
Hypophosphatemia, 6
Hypothermia, multiple transfusions and, 218
Hypotonic solutions, 11i, 14

I
Idarubicin, 225t
Ifosfamide, 225t
Immunomodulatory cytokines, 231-232
Immunotherapy, 229-232
Implantable pumps, 130i
Incompatibility, 151-152, 213
Infection, 71, 124-127, 147, 181
Infiltration, 66, 177
Infusion flow rates, calculating, 22, 23i
Infusion methods, 155-162
Infusions. See also specific therapy.
    adding drugs during, 154, 167
    administering, 163-169

Infusions (continued)
    chemotherapy. See Chemotherapy.
    continuous, 20, 21, 155, 156
    direct injection, 157, 158, 163-165
    in elderly patients, 172
    intermittent. See Intermittent infusion.
    pediatric, 170
    through secondary line, 168
    simultaneous, set-up for, 54, 55i
    vascular access port, 131-133, 134-138
Injection, direct, 15, 16, 157, 158, 163-164, 165
Insertion line, 97, 117
Interferon, 231
Interleukins, 231
Intermittent infusion, 17-19
    using piggyback method, 17, 159
    using saline lock, 18, 160, 166
    using volume-control set, 19, 161, 162i, 167
Irritants, chemotherapeutic, 240, 244-245
Isotonic solutions, 11i, 12
I.V. push, 15

J
Jugular veins, 99i, 100, 101

K
Ketone bodies, in nutritional deficiencies, 269t

L
Labeling, of I.V. bags, 24
Laminar airflow hood, 234
Leucovorin, 226t
Leukocytes, 189
Leukopenia, chemotherapy and, 254
Leuprolide, 226t
Ligament damage, peripheral I.V. therapy and, 67
Light, and drug incompatibility, 151
Lipid emulsions, in parenteral nutrition solutions, 275
Long-line catheter, 79-80, 95-96, 95i
Lung cancer, 228t
Lymphoma, 228t

M
Macrodrip, 22, 23i
Magnesium, 5
Malnutrition, protein-calorie, 260, 262
Median antebrachial vein, 29i, 32

i refers to an illustration; t refers to a table.

Medication therapy, 150, 170-182
Megestrol, 226t
Mesna, 226t
Metabolic acidosis, parenteral nutrition and, 290
Metacarpal veins, 29i, 30
Methotrexate, 225t
Metopic vein, 57i
Microdrip, 22, 23i
Micronutrients, in parenteral nutrition solutions, 273
Minerals, in parenteral nutrition solutions, 272
Mitomycin, 225t, 228t
Mitoxantrone, 225t
Mixing drugs, and drug incompatibility, 151
Monoclonal antibodies, 230t

**N**

Nausea and vomiting, chemotherapy and, 255-256
Needle, incorrect placement of, 144t
Needle gauges, 41t
Nerve damage, peripheral I.V. therapy and, 67
Nonvesicants, chemotherapeutic, 240, 244-245
Nutritional assessment, 263-269
    anthropometry in, 265-266, 265-266i
    diagnostic studies in, 267-269t
Nutritional deficiencies, 260-262

**O**

Occlusion, peripheral I.V. therapy and, 68
Oncovin, 228t
Orders, contents of, 22
Over-the-needle catheter, 37-38, 37i
Oxyhemoglobin dissociation curve, effect of multiple transfusions on, 219

**PQ**

Packed red blood cells, 186-187
Parenteral nutrition, 259-293
    discontinuing, 280
    in elderly patients, 283
    managing problems in, 280-281, 280-281t, 283-293
    in pediatric patients, 282
Parenteral nutrition solutions, 270-275
Patient-controlled analgesia, 169
Peripheral I.V. therapy, 27-76
    changing administration set in, 53

Peripheral I.V. therapy *(continued)*
    dressings in, 51, 51i, 52
    in elderly patients, 59
    infusing additive solutions in, 54, 55i
    maintaining, 49-55, 49i, 51i, 55i
    managing complications of, 60-75
    in pediatric patients, 56-58, 57i
    taping methods in, 49-50, 49i
Peripheral parenteral nutrition, 271, 278-279
Peripherally inserted central catheter, 79-80
pH, and drug incompatibility, 151
Phlebitis, 69, 178-179, 291
Phosphorus, 6
Piggyback method, for intermittent infusion, 17, 159
Plant alkaloids, chemotherapeutic, 225t
Plasma, 195, 199
Plasma fractions, 195
Plasma products, 199-202
Plasma protein incompatibility reaction, blood transfusion and, 213
Platelets, 190-191
Platinol, 228t
Pneumothorax, 122-123
Port, deeply implanted, 145t
Port migration, 144t
Potassium, 7
Potassium intoxication, multiple transfusions and, 220
Prealbumin, 269t
Prednisone, 228t
Pressure cuff, 197
Progestins, chemotherapeutic, 226t
Protein-calorie deficiencies, 260-262
Pumps, implantable, 130i

**R**

Red blood cells, 186-187, 188
Rituximab, 230t

**S**

Safety precautions, for chemotherapy, 235-239
Saline, buffered, 200
Saline lock, 18, 160, 166
Saline solution, 108
Sampling, 48, 142
Scalp vein catheter, 58
Scalp veins, in pediatric patients, 56, 57i

i refers to an illustration; t refers to a table.

Sepsis, parenteral nutrition and, 292
Short-term multilumen catheter, 85-86, 85i
Short-term single-lumen catheter, 83-84, 83i
Skin breakdown, vascular access port
    therapy and, 147
Sodium, 8
Solutions, 11-14, 11i. *See also specific type.*
  flushing, 108-109
  3:1, 274
Spasm, venous, 75, 182
Speed shock, medication therapy, 180
Stomatitis, chemotherapy and, 257
Subclavian vein, 991, 102
Syringe pump, for pediatric patients, 171
Syringe technique, for drawing blood, 113, 139

**T**

Tamoxifen, 226t
Taping I.V. site, methods for, 49-50, 49i
Temperature, and drug incompatibility, 151
Tendon damage, peripheral I.V. therapy and, 67
Testolactone, 226t
Thioguanine, 225t
Thiotepa, 225t
3:1 solution, 274
Thrombocytopenia, chemotherapy and, 258
Thrombophlébitis, 72
Thrombosis, 72, 128, 148
Total lymphocyte count, in nutritional
    deficiencies, 269t
Total nutrient admixture, 274-275
Total parenteral nutrition, 270, 276-277. *See
    also* Parenteral nutrition.
Total protein screen, in nutritional
    deficiencies, 269t
Trace elements, in parenteral nutrition
    solutions, 273
Transferrin, in nutritional deficiencies, 268t
Transfusion reactions, 196, 208-220
Transfusions, 183-220
  administering, 192-199
  blood. *See* Blood transfusion.
  cellular products and, 184-191, 194
  in elderly patients, 204
  multiple, managing reactions to, 214-220
  in pediatric patients, 203
  of plasma or plasma fractions, 195
  preparing for, 192-193

Transparent semipermeable dressing, 51, 51i
Transthyretin, in nutritional deficiencies, 269t
Triglycerides, in nutritional deficiencies, 268t
Tubing, 110, 144t
Tumor necrosis factor, 232
Tunneled catheter, 81

**U**

U method, for securing I.V. site, 49, 49i

**V**

Vascular access port, 129, 132-135, 139-141
Vascular access port implantation, 129, 130i
Vascular access port infusion
  continuous, administering, 136, 142
  discontinuing, 137
  maintaining, 134-138
  managing complications of, 143-148
  performing, 131-133
  removing noncoring needle in, 138
  selecting needle for, 131
  troubleshooting problems with, 144-145t
Vein irritation, peripheral I.V. therapy and, 74
Veins
  direct injection into, 157, 163-164
  in peripheral I.V. therapy, 28-36, 29i
  scalp, 56, 57i
  in venipuncture, 42, 46
Venipuncture, 42-48
Venipuncture devices, 37-41, 37i, 40i, 41t
  documenting insertion of, 24
  securing, 49-50, 49i
Venipuncture sites, peripheral, 28-36, 29i
Venous spasm, 75, 182
Venous thrombosis, parenteral nutrition
    and, 293
Vertical laminar airflow hood, 234
Vesicants, 175, 240, 242-243
Vinblastine, 225t
Vincristine, 225t, 228t
Vitamins, in parenteral nutrition solutions, 273
Volume-control set, 19, 161, 162i, 167

**WXYZ**

Water, in parenteral nutrition solutions, 273
White blood cells, 189
Whole blood, 184-185
Winged steel needle set, 39, 40i

i refers to an illustration; t refers to a table.